PALEO FITNESS

PRIMAL TRAINING AND NUTRITION TO GET LEAN, STRONG AND HEALTHY

DARRYL EDWARDS
WITH BRETT STEWART
AND JASON WARNER

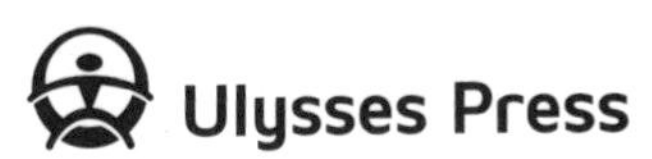

This book is dedicated to all those who have influenced, inspired and supported me on my journey to better health.
—Darryl Edwards

Published in the United States by
Ulysses Press
P.O. Box 3440
Berkeley, CA 94703
www.ulyssespress.com

ISBN13: 978-1-61243-165-9
Library of Congress Control Number 2013931800

Printed in the United States by Bang Printing

10 9 8 7 6 5 4 3 2

Recipe Contributor: Corey Irwin
Acquisitions Editor: Keith Riegert
Managing Editor: Claire Chun
Editors: Lauren Harrison, Lily Chou
Proofreader: Elyce Berrigan-Dunlop
Index: Sayre Van Young
Design and layout: what!design @ whatweb.com
Production: Jake Flaherty
Cover photographs: © Rapt Productions
Interior photographs: page 29 © Kzenon/Shutterstock.com; page 135 Darryl Edwards pushing car © Phillip Waterman
Models: Darryl Edwards, Sabrina Rose Lau, Chad Taylor

Please Note
This book conveys the authors' opinions and ideas based on their research and training, as well as each of their experiences with their clients. This book has been written and published strictly for informational and educational purposes only, and in no way should be used as a substitute for consultation with health care professionals. You should not consider educational material herein to be the practice of medicine or to replace consultation with a physician or other medical practitioner. You should always consult with your physician before altering or changing any aspect of your medical treatment and/or undertaking a diet regimen, including the guidelines as described in this book. The authors and publisher are providing you with information in this work so that you can have the knowledge and can choose, at your own risk, to act on that knowledge. The author and publisher also urge all readers to be aware of their health status and to consult health care professionals before beginning any health or diet program.

TABLE OF CONTENTS

FOREWORD

Everyone is on a "diet." Everything you see on TV, read online, browse in the latest magazines, or even spot on a subway advertisement contains the latest and greatest "secret tip" or "magic pill" or "can't-lose celebrity diet." Not only is it impossible to avoid the deluge of carefully crafted marketing messages and big-time star endorsements, it's even more difficult to make sense of it all and figure out what's right for you—not just for the next few weeks while you're "on a diet," but for the rest of your life. "On a diet" is a ludicrous phrase that refers to a finite amount of time where you diverge from consistent eating patterns and essentially make yourself miserable in order to attempt to quickly lose weight, only to put all that weight (and more) back on when you end the insanity. Lose-gain-lose-gain, yo-yo dieting isn't only unhealthy physically, it's a mental mind-scramble that leads to a distorted body image, even more confusion about how to use nutrition properly, and eventually a total disregard for healthy food choices—essentially giving up.

Nutrition and fitness combined are the most important investments that we can ever make during our lifetime, as the benefits are immediately apparent: a healthier, happier, and longer life filled with activities and adventures. The virtues of a sound mind and body have been etched in our collective consciousness since the dawn of man; even in the earliest cave drawings, humans were crudely depicted as fit and strong when they hunted mighty beasts. There wasn't a spare tire of bulging gut to be found. With all the advances humans have made in the ten thousand years since the Paleolithic era, it appears that modern man's waistline has expanded significantly as well.

Over the past decade during my journey of knowledge in nutrition, activity, adventure, functional training, fitness and endurance races, I've studied, experimented with, and written about vegetarianism, veganism, no-carb, carbohydrate manipulation, high-protein and nutrition for ultra-endurance athletes. Now, with the knowledge and guidance from one of the premiere spokespeople for Paleo fitness and nutrition, Darryl Edwards, and the tireless research and testing of my right-hand man, Jason Warner, I'm pleased to present *Paleo Fitness: A Nutrition and Training Program for Athletes on the Caveman Diet.*

This book's roots are based in sound nutritional advice and science, not a diet craze or fitness fad. The nutritional lessons we explore have existed for millennia. The functional movements are inspired by and crafted for the actions you perform every day. Using these functional movements, we'll open up an entirely new world of possibilities for your own exercise. What you'll find on these pages is more than a diet or a fitness regimen—it's a sustainable lifestyle change that can yield extremely positive results for your body and mind!

I hope you enjoy reading this book and following along with the exercises, recipes, and tips. It has been an eye-opening and exciting journey for me, and I trust it will be for you as well.

—Brett Stewart
coauthor of *The Vegan Athlete*

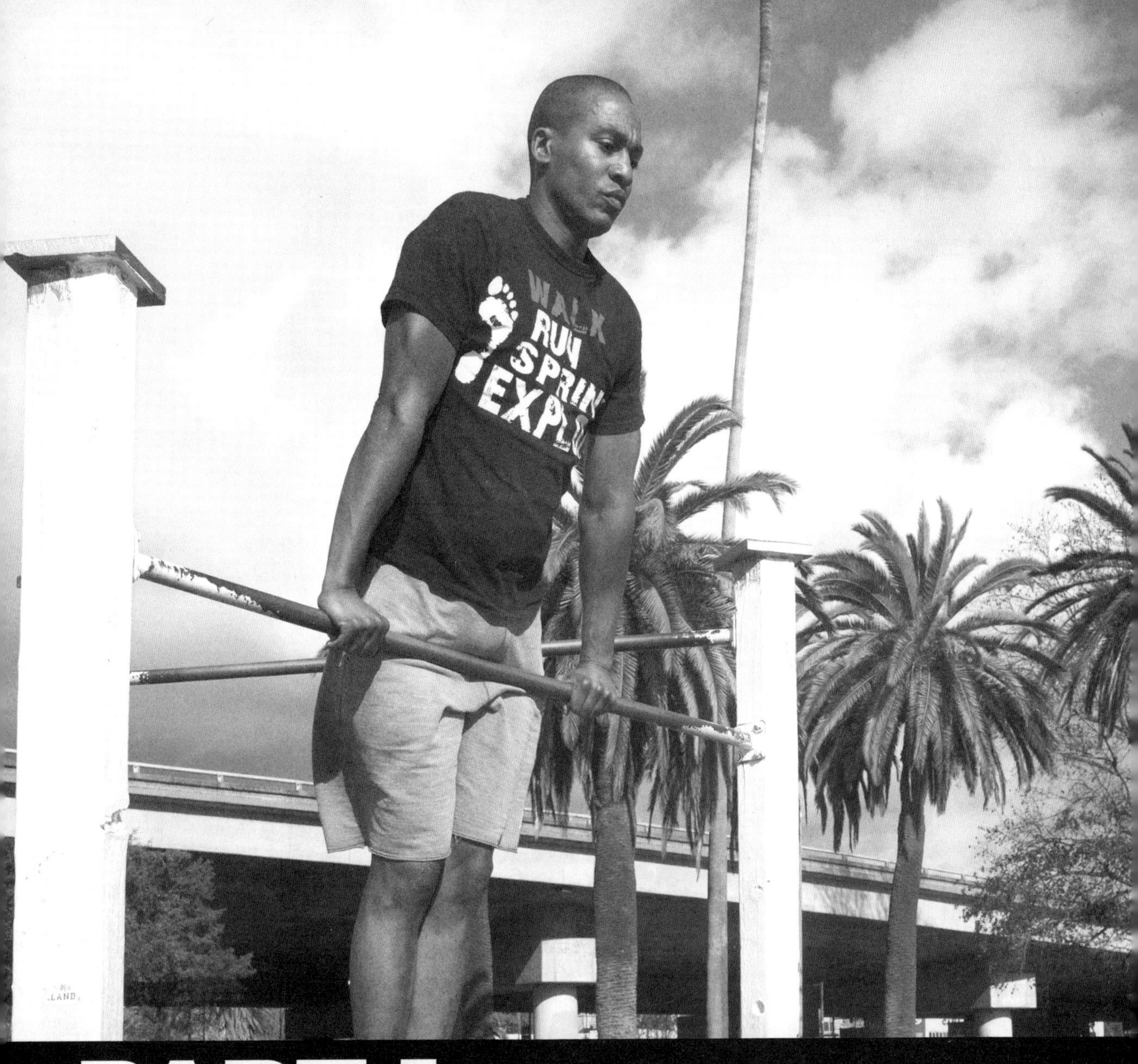

PART I: OVERVIEW

INTRODUCTION

So many people spend their health gaining wealth, and then have to spend their wealth to regain their health. —A. J. Reb Materi

Thanks to medical advances and improvements in hygiene, we're all living longer lives but are sicker than ever before. An ever-increasing majority are burdened with chronic diseases such as cardiovascular disease (heart attacks and strokes), cancers, diabetes and chronic respiratory diseases, all inextricably linked to the lifestyle choices we make.

The World Health Organization (WHO) reports that most of these noncommunicable diseases (NCDs) have a strong correlation and causation with four risk factors: tobacco use, lack of physical activity, alcohol abuse and poor nutrition. These lifestyle decisions lead to detectable physiological changes with high risk of death. Elevated blood pressure is the leading risk factor attributed to 13% of deaths globally, followed by tobacco use (9%), elevated blood glucose (6%), physical inactivity (6%) and being overweight or obese (5%). In 2008, NCDs contributed to 63% of all deaths globally. By 2030,NCDs are anticipated to cause 75% of global deaths.

One thing's for certain: Opting for a quick fix isn't the answer for the long term. Prevention has to be the ultimate goal. The good news is these risk factors are preventable and reversible.

One possible solution to getting a lean, healthy body lies with our hunter-gatherer ancestors. Anthropological evidence tells us that our Paleolithic forebears were lean, tall and athletic and avoided the chronic diseases that plague us today. By looking backward to move forward, we can reintroduce key elements of our ancestors' lifestyle—better food choices, appropriate physical activity and stress management will mitigate the risks associated with the development of chronic disease. Going back to the better aspects of even a generation or two ago would lead to better health today.

I used to believe (and the contemporary viewpoints offered in most circles still suggest) that the answer to improving one's health is to clear the residue from the past, take a deep breath, refocus and continue. There are times when your computer doesn't respond to tweaking, and the only way to accomplish the desired result of a healthy PC is to "reboot" it. As humans, we may decide on a detox to wipe the slate clean; however, a "reboot" just like a "detox" works only in the short term. The only way to ensure long-term benefit is to perform an "upgrade." An upgrade is what I'm mandating here: an "upgrade" of our mindset to encompass a lifestyle change. *Paleo Fitness* should not be seen as a quick fix but as an effective method to kick-start a new attitude toward food, activity and life.

According to food behavior expert Brian Wansink in his book *Mindless Eating: Why We Eat More Than We Think*, we make nearly 200 food-related decisions every day, 90% of which are subconscious. David Kessler elaborates on this further in the book *The End of Overeating: Taking Control of the Insatiable American Appetite*. To summarize both Wansink and Kessler, we overeat because of signals in our environment.

We have a basic instinctive drive to seek out high-calorie, energy-dense foods in times of plenty to ensure survival once food becomes scarce. Unfortunately, most of the foods manufactured today are energy dense but nutritionally void. If we only eat these foods occasionally, then arguably there's minimal impact, but the abundance at every opportunity makes them difficult to resist. It's difficult to make the right food choices with all of the many distractions available to us, especially when it's part of our genetic blueprint to react this way.

In *Paleo Fitness*, we'll share my journey as a personal trainer, movement coach, and fitness and health explorer who, like countless others, has transformed his strength, fitness and well-being since adopting a Paleolithic lifestyle. We'll suggest uncomplicated strategies that lead to better decision making for health. We'll also share deliciously practical Paleo recipes created by an award-winning chef that are extremely nutritious, delivering examples of food for an individual to get lean, strong and healthier while following the beginner, intermediate or advanced fitness plans included in the appendix.

Food Myths

There's so much conflicting information out there about diet, nutrition and exercise. Pseudoscience, myths and old wives' tales abound and the public is quite rightly often skeptical and confused. What we hear is often ambiguous and confusing. What are we to believe?

Which of the following statements do you think are true about diet and exercise?

- Eating too much fat causes you to store fat.
- Eating high levels of fat causes you to burn fat.
- Eating carbohydrates after a certain time of the day will drive your body to store the calories as excess fat.
- Eating excessive carbohydrates at any time will cause your body to store the calories as fat.
- We can be overweight and healthy.
- Being overweight is unhealthy.
- Not eating breakfast will cause your body to enter starvation mode so you're more likely to gain weight.
- Eating a high-protein meal at breakfast means you'll be less likely to snack during the day.
- Exercising on an empty stomach will cause you to burn fat for energy.
- Exercising on an empty stomach will cause you to release the stress hormone cortisol, which will break down body tissue, preventing fat loss and promoting muscle wastage.
- Genetics determine whether you have a slow or fast metabolism and there's nothing you can do about it.
- Lifestyle has more impact on our metabolism than genetics do.
- To lose weight, you must eat less and exercise more.
- To lose weight, you must eat less fat.
- Our metabolisms slow down as we age, so we gain weight as we age.
- Our metabolism is constant throughout our lives; a lack of activity as we age causes us to put on weight.
- Exercise in your fat-burning zone by doing cardio activities to lose weight.

Overweight or Obese?

Overweight refers to an individual weighing more than his or her recommended healthy weight. *Obesity* is a medical condition in which excess body fat has accumulated to the point where it will have an adverse effect on health and life expectancy, and will increase the risk of contracting other life-threatening diseases, including cancer, heart disease, type 2 diabetes, and high blood pressure.

The worldwide obesity epidemic is a relatively new phenomenon. The Organization for Economic Cooperation and Development (OECD), in the report "Obesity and the Economics of Prevention: Fit Not Fat," stated that in 1980 obesity rates were well below 10%. Since then, the rates have doubled or tripled in the world's 33 richest countries.

In 2008, 1.5 billion adults over 20 years old were overweight, globally. Of these, over 200 million men and nearly 300 million women were obese. In comparison, there are 870 million people who are chronically hungry.

A recent report by Trust for America's Health and the Robert Wood Johnson Foundation forecasts that more than half of Americans will be obese by 2030.

- Build muscle to burn fat by doing strength and resistance exercises.
- High-intensity workouts will blitz body fat and build muscle.
- Eat whatever you want as long you do enough exercise.
- Eat the right foods at the right times to maintain your ideal weight.
- Eat one very large meal a day, then fast for the rest of the day to burn fat.
- Eat three square meals a day just like your grandmother used to do.
- Eat five to six times a day so as not to overload the digestive system.
- Eat little and often, grazing like a cow, to keep blood sugar levels constant.
- Eat breakfast like a king, lunch like a prince, and dinner like a pauper.
- Detox every two weeks to rid the body of toxins and lose weight in the process.
- Don't eat carbs after midday, 2 p.m, 4 p.m.—or is it supposed to be after 6 p.m.?

It's all far too confusing! The health benefits of certain foods one week seem to be contradicted by follow-up research the next. Eggs, for example, are back in favor after years of concern about dietary cholesterol; current research shows that eggs reduce "bad" LDL cholesterol levels in the blood based on the nutrient choline, and they actively decrease blood pressure. Other research states that dietary cholesterol has no impact on serum cholesterol levels in the body. It's a recipe for confusion and often leaves us with more questions than answers.

Each successive post-war generation has enjoyed an increasingly sedentary lifestyle, accompanied by an increase in obesity. Obesity, already associated with high-income countries in the West, is now increasingly prevalent in middle- and low-income countries, too. General efforts aimed at helping people lose weight have so far proven ineffective. Obesity triggers many secondary health issues, a primary concern for public health organizations worldwide.

The Diet Smorgasbord

I personally dislike the associations around the word "diet." Why? Because it usually suggests something that's temporary. It's often used when referring to the eating habits of people who restrict and limit foods to change their body shape for the short term. A "diet" conjures up a punishing regimen requiring significant self-sacrifice that isn't something you plan to do for the rest of your life. But when we investigate the origins of the word *diet* from the ancient Greek word *diaita* or from the Latin *diaeta*, it means "the prescribed way of life." This is how we should approach Paleo nutrition—not as a limitation but an enhancement to one's way of living.

Let's take a look at some of the diet choices available before we put the Paleo diet into context.

THE LOWS: These are diets based on eating lower proportions of a macronutrient (fat, protein or carbohydrate). Common examples include low-fat diets like the Pritikin Diet and the Dean Ornish Diet. Low-carbohydrate diets, like the Atkins Diet, Carb-Buster and the South Beach Diet, are increasingly seen as effective ways to lose weight in the short term. Low-protein diets are primarily designed for those diagnosed with kidney or liver disease. "The Lows" also include meal plans aimed to significantly reduce calorie intake for short periods of time, such as the 500 Calorie a Day Diet, the Cambridge Diet and Medifast.

THE HIGHS: These are diets based on eating relatively high proportions of macronutrients, such as the high-protein diets used by bodybuilders and weightlifters on a long-term basis to build lean muscle mass and burn fat in conjunction with a mostly anaerobic, resistance-based workout. There are high-carbohydrate diets, like the 80/10/10 Diet or the McDougall Diet, which aim to totally eliminate fats. On the other end of the spectrum, high-fat diets usually fall into the category of ketogenic diets, which are used primarily as treatment for refractory epilepsy in young children, as well as morbid obesity, type 2 diabetes, Alzheimer's disease, Parkinson's disease and cancer. These diets force the body to burn fats rather than carbohydrates as energy.

The list of other "popular" nutritional plans goes on. There's the Zone Diet, the Blood Type Diet, acid-alkaline diets, Glycemic Index diets, mono food diets, vegetarianism, veganism, the fruitarian diet, the macrobiotic diet and even the breatharian diet. The latter is based on the belief that the only energy humans need for survival are oxygen and sunlight.

The Western Pattern Diet, otherwise known as the Standard American Diet (SAD), typifies the diet of affluence in developed countries and is increasingly adopted in developing countries. This diet is rich in highly refined carbohydrates, high levels of dissolved sugar in the form of sweetened drinks, high levels of salt and artificial flavorings, poor-quality fats, processed meat and a lack of fresh fruit, fish, meat and vegetables. This diet is linked to everything from poor behavior in children to depression and increased risk of lifestyle diseases.

The lack of sustainable weight-loss success certainly isn't due to a lack of knowledge. It's likely we have more information available on food and nutrition than at any time in human history. Most of the information we rely on has one fundamental flaw: It ignores nature and the historical context of mankind. The choices we make now need to be considered on that basis. When we deviate from nature and our heritage as hunter-gatherers, we do so to our detriment.

Just forget about dieting and focus on your diet.

From nearly the first word to the last, this book documents not just one but several journeys into learning about the Paleo lifestyle, diet, fitness plan and movements to profoundly change the individuals who have and will take this trip. The vast majority of the book follows Darryl's research and development of training plans for himself and his clients that put the "fun" back in functional fitness—with some remarkable results. Jason changed his body composition and way of looking at nutrition, which potentially prevented developing diabetes. Brett developed a much deeper appreciation for functional fitness that led to him becoming a better athlete and trainer, and even helped to spawn his writing career. Corey Irwin, nutritional expert and recipe developer, spent hundreds of hours creating and testing the recipes you'll find in this book, along the way modifying her own nutritional intake to reap the benefits of the Paleo diet.

Whether you're interested in learning more about following the Paleo lifestyle, beginning to embrace Paleo nutrition and functional cross-training into your daily routine or are already practicing Paleo, this book features plenty of in-depth nutritional and fitness information that you'll find extremely helpful to achieve your goals.

The authors' results have been nothing short of eye-opening. Incorporating all or a some of the Paleo lifestyle that you'll find in this book can have a positive effect on your health and overall well-being.

WHAT IS THE PALEOLITHIC DIET?

The Paleolithic diet, also known as the Stone Age, caveman, ancestral or hunter-gatherer diet, is a modern interpretation of what our ancestors ate in Paleolithic (Stone Age) times as hunter-gatherers.

You may have heard of the Paleo diet from a friend or relative, or read about it in a book or magazine. Many people try Paleo in hopes of enhancing their overall health, to prevent and fight disease or to change their body composition. It's common for individuals to reduce their body fat percentage and maintain an ideal weight relatively quickly, usually kick-started with a 30-day challenge of some kind. These are all good reasons to try the Paleo diet, but many people stick with it even after they've accomplished their short-term goals.

The idea of a modern diet based on ancient ancestry goes back to a book published in 1938 entitled *Nutrition and Physical Degeneration: A Comparison of Primitive and Modern Diets and Their Effects* by Dr. Weston Price, who traveled extensively across the globe and observed that whenever modern diets were taken on by non-Westernized groups of people, their health plummeted. Since Price's research, many other scientists have similarly found that a diet more in keeping with what our ancestors ate keeps populations healthier.

The Evolution of Research: Documenting the Paleolithic Diet

In the mid-1970s, gastroenterologist Walter Voegtlin was one of the first to mention the relationship between improving human health and following a Paleo-type diet in the book *The Stone Age Diet: Based on In-Depth Studies of Human Ecology and the Diet of Man.*

In 1985, a landmark research paper published in the *New England Journal of Medicine* entitled "Paleolithic Nutrition: A consideration of its nature and current implications" by Dr. S. Boyd Eaton and Dr. Melvin Konner showed that modern humans are almost identical to our Paleolithic ancestors in terms of genetics—a mere 0.02% genetic difference. This genetic makeup is largely discordant with life today.

In the late 1980s, this idea took on mainstream medical significance with the book *The Paleolithic Prescription* by Dr. S. Boyd Eaton, Dr. Melvin Konner and Dr. Marjorie Shostak. It linked the importance of physical activity and the proportions of nutrients in a Paleolithic diet.

In the 1990s, the Swedish medical doctor and scientist Staffan Lindeberg published the "Kitava Study" based on his work with present-day hunter-gatherers in Papua New Guinea and established that they didn't suffer from stroke, ischemic heart disease, diabetes, obesity or hypertension based on their diet.

First published in 2000, Ray Audette's *NeanderThin: Eat Like a Caveman to Achieve a Lean, Strong, Healthy Body* spoke about eating a "caveman" diet, documenting what early humans ate and the diseases they avoided. He also discussed what happened to us post-agriculture.

In 2002, Dr. Loren Cordain, a professor in health and exercise science at the University of Colorado, did a batch of research work in the 1990s that led to the first edition of his book *The Paleo Diet*, which introduced the role of chronic inflammation as the underlying reason for many lifestyle diseases. Cordain updated his works with *The Paleo Answer* in 2012.

In 2011, research biochemist Robb Wolf covered biochemistry, genetics, and anthropology with updated topics in the book *The Paleolithic Solution.*

The Paleolithic era is assumed to cover over 2.5 million years, ending around 20,000 years ago. The foods of this period consisted of lean meats, fowl, fish, eggs, vegetables, nuts and fruit. It didn't include sugar, grains, dairy products, legumes (beans), salt, or processed and artificial foods.

Researchers examining health from an anthropological perspective have found that our ancestors were lean, tall, strong, fit and in good health. After taking into account the daily risks of being eaten by predators, short life expectancy at birth, poor hygiene or contracting infectious diseases, life expectancy was as good as the present day. They were also free of the chronic lifestyle diseases that afflict us today. There's evidence that not only were our ancestors' periods of intense activity beneficial, diet also was key to their health.

The Science behind the Diet

There are many studies that support this modern take on the Paleolithic diet. One study widely reported in the British press in 2008 was the trial run by the Karolinska Institutet in Sweden, published in the *European Journal of Clinical Nutrition.*

Subjects were only allowed to eat fruit, vegetables, lean meat, fish, and nuts. All beans, grains (wheat, rice) alcohol, sugar, and juices were banned. In just three weeks the subjects lost an average of 5 pounds, their waist circumference reduced by 0.2 inches, they saw a 5% decrease in blood pressure and had 72% lower levels of a blood-clotting agent that could cause heart attacks and strokes.

Dr. Per Wandell noted at the time, "Short-term intervention with a Paleolithic diet in healthy volunteers showed some favorable effects on cardiovascular risk factors."

When did this all change?

AGRICULTURAL REVOLUTION: The Paleolithic diet of fresh fruits, vegetables, meats and fish remained consistent until 10,000 years or so ago when we started to leave behind our hunter-gatherer past. Instead of consuming foods we would typically hunt, gather or scavenge, we began to cultivate the soil, grow crops (including previously inedible or difficult to digest grains) and domesticate animals for livestock. Although our world has changed radically in the last 10,000 years, the human genome has hardly changed since then.

INDUSTRIAL REVOLUTION: In the 18th to 19th centuries, a shift to industry brought about significant improvements in agricultural productivity, and machinery replaced much of the work previously done by manual labor.

FAST-FOOD REVOLUTION: The advances in manufacturing, technology and food science of the last 50 years have made mass-produced food based around grain, sugar, low-quality fat and man-made substances the norm. With the supersize- and value-meal culture introduced in the U.S. in the late 1960s and Western Europe in the 1980s, larger meals were produced more quickly and cheaply than before. Portion sizes are up to five times larger than in the 1950s, and the average soda, then of 7 ounces, can now be up to 64 ounces!

LOW-FAT REVOLUTION: Fat is an essential nutrient; however, even with this knowledge and increased availability of low-fat produce over the last few decades, there has not been a corresponding downward trend in obesity levels.

Genetically our bodies are virtually identical to our hunter-gatherer ancestors in terms of biochemistry and physiology. In the last 200 years, developments in agriculture and industry have changed how we cultivate and obtain foods. The rise of fast food and other convenience products has changed what we eat. Also, fundamental social norms have evolved. When I was growing up in the 1970s, eating on the streets or on public transport was something that was frowned upon. Nowadays this is far more accepted and indeed encouraged given the number of food outlets that don't even provide seating. We have far more options and opportunities to eat on the go. Any yearning for food must be immediately satisfied with snacks (or mini-meals) rather than waiting for the next available meal time.

Our bodies adapted during the Paleolithic time to the environment and conditions of that time. If what we ate to develop, thrive and survive then is removed from us and replaced with nutrient-deficient foods such as those so prevalent in modern society, then as human beings we're bound to suffer. One key driving theory for the Paleo diet is that modern humans' digestive systems aren't designed to handle the refined sugars, grains, legumes,and dairy products that are now commonplace in the Western diet.

There's more awareness about the relationship between the food we eat and the risks associated with the lifestyle diseases of obesity, diabetes, cancer, heart disease and strokes. The objective of the Paleo lifestyle is to pick the critical aspects of Paleolithic life that make a positive difference. We don't want to turn a blind eye to the medical and technological advances that have improved human health and well-being, but integrating the best of our ancestral inheritance with the best of the present enables us to achieve optimal wellness.

The idea is to use this Paleo template as a starting point, weigh the options in terms of the health risks when we stray from this road map and to look at food in the context of nutrient quality. The basic principle of a Paleolithic diet is straightforward. When deciding to eat a particular food, ask yourself: Is this something that would be edible in the absence of modern technology and agriculture?

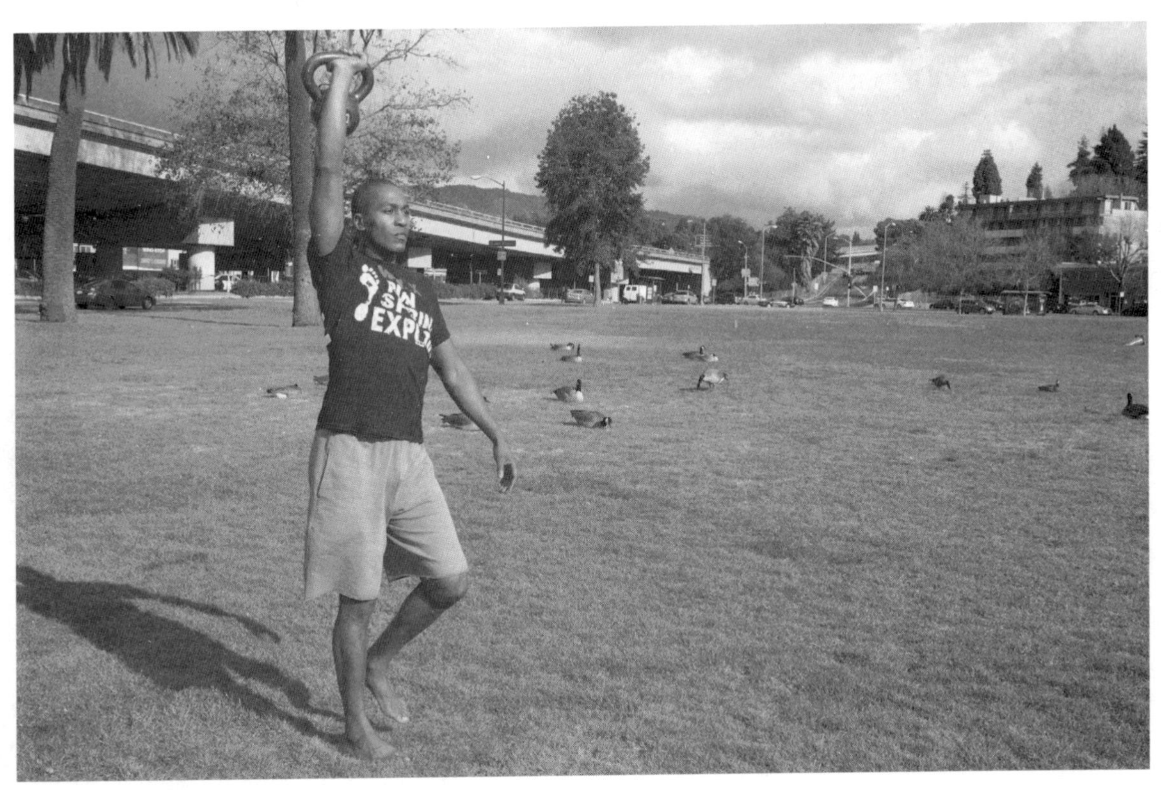

Some Benefits of the Paleo Diet

Based on clinical trials, personal observation and a wide array of anecdotal evidence, the Paleo lifestyle has a positive impact on many of the chronic diseases plaguing Western society. It can:

- Improve insulin sensitivity, as more foods are eaten with lower glycemic loads.
- Reduce hypertension by reducing sodium (salt) intake, resulting in a better sodium/potassium ratio.
- Reduce body fat and improve body composition.
- Improve bone density through increased levels of micronutrient intake, as well as improve bioavailability of the required minerals.
- Reduce inflammation by raising the body's anti-inflammatory profile through an improved omega 3:6 ratio (inflammation is a significant risk factor for a number of modern diseases).
- Allow remission and management of certain diseases (such as celiac disease, type 1 and type 2 diabetes, rheumatoid arthritis, Crohn's disease, irritable bowel syndrome and ulcerative colitis) without drugs.
- Reduce exposure to food toxins and pollutants through the choosing of organic and naturally reared products.
- Improve digestion with better gut flora.
- Improve nutrient absorption (for example, vitamins A, D, E and K are fat-soluble vitamins; low-fat diets reduce the absorption of these vitamins).
- Improve sleep quality by eliminating or reducing beverages containing caffeine and alcohol, which affect the quantity and quality of deep and REM sleep.

What about Activity?

Today, most of us are less active than our parents and grandparents were and far less active than hunter-gatherer people of the past. Recent studies show that inactivity is linked to poor health. Exercise protects us from depression and a wide array of illnesses, and even boosts memory. Sedentary people have a 35% greater risk of developing high blood pressure (hypertension) than those who exercise regularly.

Hypertension is often termed the "silent killer" because many people are unaware they have the condition. In late 2012, the medical journal *The Lancet* published large-scale research that identified hypertension as the world's biggest killer. Suffering from hypertension in the long term can affect the:

- heart, causing congestive heart failure
- brain, causing strokes
- kidneys, causing kidney damage and failure
- vascular system (blood vessels), causing peripheral arterial disease and aneurysms
- eyes, causing eye damage and blindness.

Feed Your Body, Feed Your Mind

What we eat affects not only how we look and perform, but most significantly how we think and feel. From birth, every piece of food and drink we ingest becomes a part of us—a source of energy to the estimated 30 to 50 trillion cells that make up the human body. These nutrients are delivered via the blood through the extensive capillary network that serves all the cells of the body.

Food is something we can often take for granted. We don't take time to consider its preparation, its source, or the benefits of real (as opposed to fake) food. We eat artificial foods created by chemists, marketed as better substitutes for the real thing. If we follow the Paleo lifestyle, we eat whole foods in the forms that will satisfy our bodies and our minds.

BEING PALEO: DARRYL'S STORY

Growing up in the '70s, I was an active child—we all were. After school, on weekends and during school holidays we would explore the outside world and play. There was one instruction given to us by mother, "Be back home for dinner!" We didn't have much choice about what to eat. You ate what you were given. Fortunately, what we were given was usually home-cooked, fresh food. We rarely snacked between meals. We drank water most of the time and a soda drink was a once-a-week treat.

I enjoyed being active and participating in sports. I was pretty much average at everything I attempted, a jack of all trades and a master of none. My father was a martial arts fan, and he would take my brother and me to the movie theater for the late-night showing of Chinese kung fu movies on the weekends. I took up Shotokan and Wado Ryu karate and Kung Tao kung fu, competing for several years until my mid-teens.

Unfortunately, once I left school, my lifestyle changed radically. Activity was something I would do on a rare occasion. In college, food was about convenience, not health. The fact that I could eat whatever food I wanted, whenever I wanted, was a bonus to me.

The situation didn't change once I started my career working in IT. My diet for most of my twenties was the stereotypical diet of choice for a computer programmer: fast-food, sweets and any beverage that wasn't water. During this time I never had an issue with my weight; in fact, I was pretty skinny for most of my late teens and early twenties even though I was eating as much as I wanted. I put this down to "good genes" and a super-fast metabolism. I would join the gym every summer to try and "bulk up" for the summer holidays with little success—without any irony I put that down to "bad genes" and a super-fast metabolism.

At the end of my twenties into my early thirties, I and others noticed the spare tire starting to appear around my middle, and I reluctantly decided to focus on making better food choices and became a regular gym rat. I prescribed to the UK government's guidelines for a healthy, low-fat diet: five portions of fruit and vegetables a day, lots of whole grains, occasional red meat, fish and dairy. I also drank whey protein shakes, took supplements and followed the guidance in fitness and bodybuilding magazines. I tried a wide variety of gym classes but didn't stick with any for more than a few weeks. Motivation was difficult and results often fleeting. I felt and looked older than my years.

By my mid-thirties, I noticed that whatever I did I couldn't get rid of the "middle-age" spread. I put this down to my age, falling short in my diet, and not working hard enough in the gym. I attempted cardio classes and ran longer distances as a way to lose fat. I also tried calorie restriction and other diets with limited success. The results were never satisfactory.

The turning point came when I had no choice but to focus on my health. I was diagnosed with iron-deficiency anemia, living with moderate hypertension of 140/100, low levels of HDL "good" cholesterol and 26% body fat. I also suffered from chronic seborrheic dermatitis, a skin condition that caused embarrassment when I ventured outside. I felt weak and lethargic, and suffered from insomnia. I endured lower back pain and would often encounter excruciating knee pain when taking part in most activities. I even began to wear knee supports to walk short distances and to walk up stairs.

It was at this point I began to look at alternative approaches to health and fitness. I began doing shorter high-intensity workouts, weighing and measuring my foods, and lifting weights to get stronger. This was a significant improvement to all of the previous attempts I had tried, but there was still something fundamentally missing. I now realize the diet and fitness plans I had tried before were not holistic enough and were far too complicated. I didn't recognize the importance of the kinds of foods that we were designed to eat. I attempted to thrive on inadequate sleep and didn't pay attention to managing stress.

I first read about the Paleolithic diet in 2003 in Loren Cordain's book *The Paleo Diet.* I was initially skeptical. Re-reading the book several times before putting it to the test, it was a couple of years before I decided to take it seriously. The only way to evaluate this fairly was to be strict. I noticed positive changes within seven days and a significant transformation in one month, with my blood pressure and cholesterol levels improving dramatically.

At this point, I decided that if Paleo nutrition improved my health, then shouldn't I investigate back-to-basics fitness methods to improve my well-being, too? This success prompted me to qualify as a personal trainer and clinical nutritionist so I could help others who faced similar health conditions.

Several years later, after continuing to eat and move in this way, my body fat now averages 10%, the spare tire has disappeared, my blood pressure is now a healthy 108/70, my dermatitis has improved without using a topical steroid cream and I'm no longer iron-deficient anemic. My resting heart rate is an "athletic" 38 beats per minute. I'm stronger and fitter now in my forties than at any other period of my life. No more back or knee pain, increased energy levels, and a renewed since of vitality. Other biomarkers of health such as cholesterol, blood triglycerides, fasting glucose, vitamin and mineral levels and many other parameters are within normal and/or optimal ranges, which had not been the case before. Based on this evidence, there was no going back.

I realize now that I had spent many years previously doing what most of us do, what I call the "chicken flight"—an approach to fitness and health in which we enjoy short and high bursts of achievement that are inevitably followed by crashes to the ground. Even fitness experts are changing their diet and workout program every few weeks or months and telling you that now they have the answer. How are we supposed to succeed if the experts are changing tack on a regular basis? They may obtain quick aesthetic wins for a six-pack "before and after" photo shoot, but they lack long-term consistency.

Rest assured, my journey with the Paleo lifestyle isn't about a series of quick wins—this is a commitment for life.

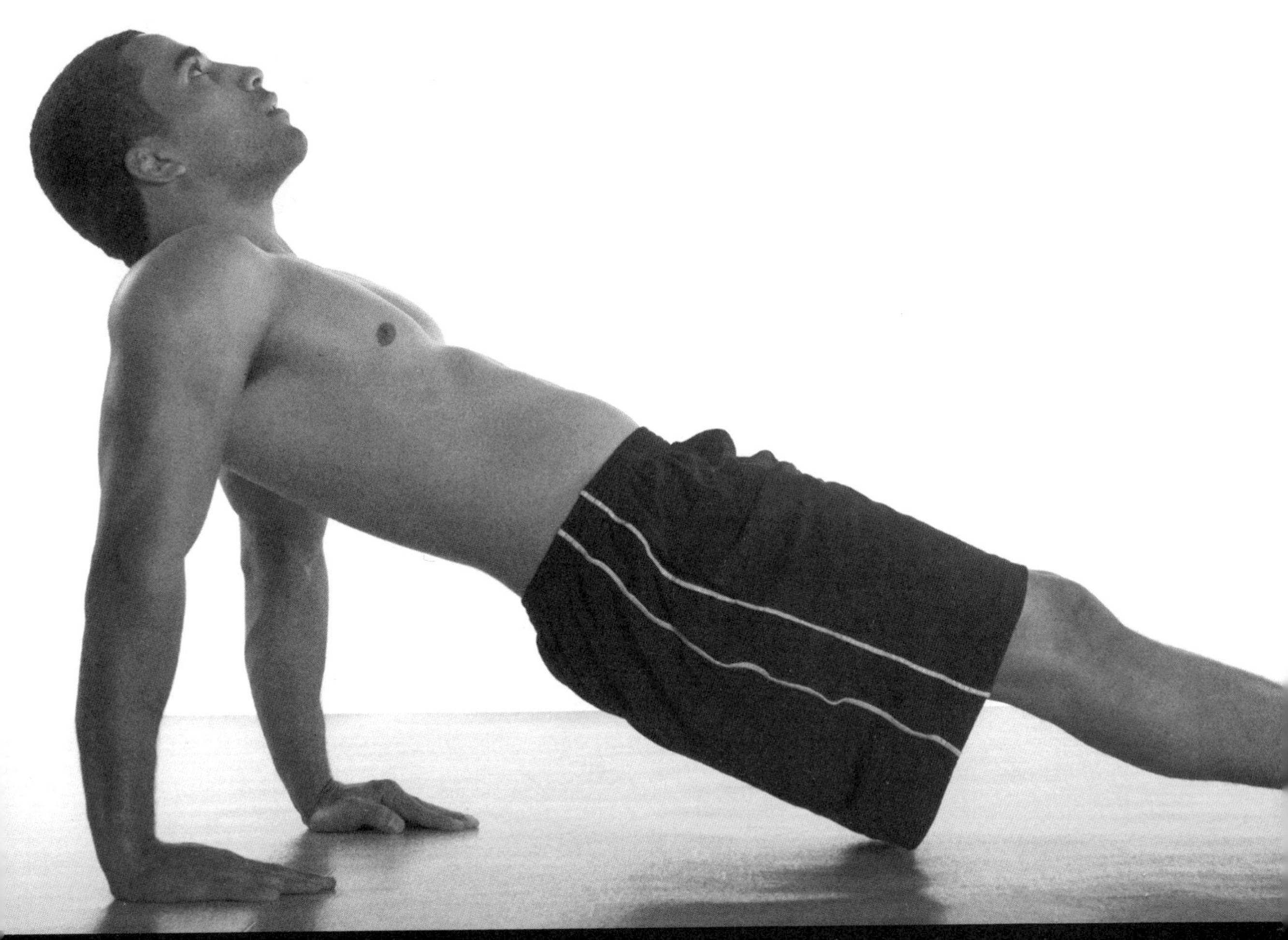

PART II: PALEO NUTRITION

FOOD FOR THE MODERN CAVEMAN

The Paleolithic diet is only a template, not a doctrine. It's a guide to help us navigate the challenges we face with modern foods that our bodies have not adapted to. The core tenet is to avoid grains, sugars, dairy and artificial/processed foods and replace them with high-quality meat, fish, eggs and vegetables whenever possible. Note that this means it's not possible to be vegan or strict vegetarian and follow the Paleo lifestyle. There are nutrients from muscle meat, organ meat and fish that aren't available from vegetarian sources.

The following list isn't exhaustive and should be used as a base platform that will ensure you make healthier food choices more often than not.

Examples of Preferred Foods

Note that for maximum health and fitness benefits, it's ideal to choose organic and free-range, naturally raised foods. The nutrient content is higher, with fewer toxins and contaminants.

MEATS: Organic, preferably grass-fed meats like beef, lamb and game such as buffalo and venison, as well as organic organ meats (liver, kidneys, etc., but only from trusted sources such as farmer's markets; make stock from leftover bones). The higher price for these high-quality meats is worth it. Grass-fed meats have a better ratio of omega-6 to omega-3 polyunsaturated fats than grain-fed meats, and organic free-range are less likely to be fed growth hormones and antibiotics.

EGGS: Preferably from pastured, free-range chickens

POULTRY: Including pastured, organic, free-range chicken, duck and turkey

FISH AND SEAFOOD: Wild-caught varieties, including salmon, sardines, cod, mackerel, trout, oysters, mussels, etc.; farmed variants are less nutritious

VEGETABLES: Organic and in-season produce, including kale, asparagus, artichokes, broccoli, cauliflower, Brussels sprouts, cabbage, lettuce, carrots, celery, cucumbers, garlic, lettuce, spinach, mushrooms, onions, turnips and watercress

NUTS: Such as almonds, Brazil nuts, walnuts, chestnuts, hazelnuts, pecans, macadamia nuts, etc. Remember—peanuts are legumes, not nuts, so they should be avoided.

FRUITS: Such as avocados, apples, olives, apricots, coconuts, dates, berries, citrus fruits, peaches, pears, grapes, melon, etc.

OIL, FOR DRESSING: Extra-virgin olive oil or walnut oil

OIL, FOR COOKING: Extra-virgin/virgin coconut oil, avocado oil

FATS, HEALTHY: Avocados, olives, coconut milk

CONDIMENTS/SEASONINGS: Herbs and spices (coriander, thyme, paprika, garlic, onions, etc.) but NO SALT

BEVERAGES: Mainly water—it's the body's most essential nutrient and makes up a significant proportion of our total body weight. Water is required by all other nutrients, chemicals, and bodily processes to travel and interact. Also acceptable are unsweetened green tea and unsweetened herbal teas like peppermint, chamomile and other non-fruit teas. Coconut water, a natural isotonic beverage, is also a great choice.

Examples of Foods to Avoid

Avoiding the following foods will make positive, detectable improvements to your health.

SUGARS: Additional sugar added to foods (such as fructose, dextrose, sucrose, high-fructose corn syrup, maltodextrin, sorbitol, xylitol) or artificial additives/substitutes; candy and sweets

GRAINS: Whole-grain or refined wheat (bread, cookies, cakes, pastry, pasta), rye, corn/maize, oats, and all other grains (including granola, millet, rice, quinoa, buckwheat, spelt, chia seeds, etc.)

MILK: All dairy products like butter, cheese, cream, whey, curds, yogurt, etc.

LEGUMES: Beans, pulses (includes soy and peanuts), etc.

POTATOES AND CASSAVA.

CONDIMENTS: Salt, vinegar, yeast

BEVERAGES: Black tea, coffee, alcohol; carbonated, sweetened (naturally or otherwise), diet, zero or low-calorie drinks; fruit and vegetable juices (which don't include any of the fibrous parts of the whole fruit or vegetable, meaning they have an increased amount of sugar)

PREPARED MEALS: Avoid all packed, pre-prepared, to-go, and ready-made meals, as most of these will contain wheat/dairy in some form and lots of additives.

PROCESSED FOODS: Do you fail to recognize one or more of the ingredients on the label without requiring a PhD in chemistry? Even though it's supposed to be natural? Then it's best to avoid.

DRIED FRUIT: Should be avoided or consumed in very small quantities because the sugar levels can be extremely high. For example, fresh mango has 15% total sugar, while dried mango has 74%, about as much as a piece of candy.

SOY, SOY MILK OR ANYTHING CONTAINING SOY PRODUCTS: There are numerous clinical and epidemiological studies that link soy to thyroid dysfunction, digestive disorders, reproductive disorders and cancer.

INDUSTRIALIZED TRANS FATS: Hydrogenated or partially hydrogenated vegetable oils found in baked goods and fried foods

VEGETABLE/SEED OILS AND SPREADS: Sunflower oil, vegetable oil, margarine, etc.

SMOOTHIES: Fruit and vegetable smoothies are packed with vitamins and minerals but can have a considerable negative impact on blood sugar levels because they have significantly less fiber than the whole fruit or vegetable. A smoothie can even contain more sugar than a can of soda!

MEAL REPLACEMENT BARS: Cereal, protein, snack or meal replacement bars of any kind

Examples of Foods to Eat in Moderation

Bananas, dense starchy tubers such as yams, sweet potatoes, butternut squash, etc., are good options for post-workout nutrition if you're lean and active. However, limit these if you're trying to lose body fat or suffer from diseases such as type 2 diabetes or hypertension.

Nuts like walnuts, almonds, Brazil nuts, and macadamia nuts are fine, but be careful with your quantities. They're easy to eat in significant amounts and given their high omega-6 to omega-3 ratios they can be pro-inflammatory in large doses. Make sure you avoid nuts that have mold; aflatoxins formed by certain molds are highly toxic and potent carcinogens (cancer-causing agents).

What's the Deal with Non-Paleo Foods?

Nature has given all species, both animals and plants, a set of defenses against predation, though not all are as clear as we may think. Not all plants have prickly thorns to protect them. However, there are other ways a plant can defend itself through its chemical constitution. Grains, legumes and even tomatoes contain chemicals designed to protect them from being eaten or to remain intact while obtaining nutrients from the host as they pass through the digestive tract. Some of these proteins are broken down by cooking, sprouting and fermenting, but others are resistant to these procedures, which leads to gut irritation and inflammation.

These defensive food substances can affect us acutely (immediately) through allergic reaction, intolerance or neurotoxin or chronically (through longer-term exposure), leading to autoimmune issues and systemic inflammation, causing disease. These compounds are anti-nutrients. It's beyond the scope of this book to cover these anti-nutrients in detail, but a basic understanding will assist you as to the "whys" of avoiding certain foods. Let's consider a few of the key culprits and some of the associated issues.

GLUTEN: All grains have similar proteins and are known to cause autoimmune issues, gastrointestinal damage and leaky gut. Gluten, found primarily in wheat but also in spelt, barley, rye and oats, blocks absorption of vitamins and alters good gut bacteria, leading to an increased risk of yeast and bacterial infections. Grains and legumes have traditionally been soaked overnight, which reduces mineral-binding phytates and enzyme-inhibitors to reduce the risk of these problems. The soaking also helps to pre-digest the food, causing less impact to the GI tract. However, instead of trying to improve the nutrient quality of less beneficial sources of carbohydrates, focus on substituting with healthier fruits and vegetables instead.

LECTINS: Lectins are proteins found in plants such as grains, seeds and legumes, as well as those in the nightshade family (such as the tomato and potato), in order to protect the seed. Lectins get stuck to the intestine and are detected as foreign invaders by the immune system. This can lead to leaky gut, other autoimmune issues and insulin resistance. Research has shown that lectins found in other plants are harmless, but some lectins found in grains, legumes and members of the nightshade family are harmful to humans.

PHYTATES: Contained in legumes like beans and peas, phytates bind to minerals such as zinc, iron, calcium, potassium and magnesium in the GI tract and extract these from the body, meaning they affect the absorption of these micronutrients and can lead to deficiency of them in the body.

SAPONINS: These are a family of toxins commonly found in potatoes and other nightshade vegetables. They bind cholesterol molecules with gut cell membranes. This new molecule increases intestinal permeability, or leaky gut. They also develop inflammatory cytokine production, leading to insulin resistance.

PROTEASE INHIBITORS: Found in soy and other legumes, these block the efficiency of protein enzymes and interfere with the breakdown of proteins into amino acids, affecting the absorption of protein.

ARTIFICIAL SWEETENERS: Artificial sweeteners are no-calorie or low-calorie substitutes used by the food industry. Some sweeteners such as sucralose are an incredible 600 times sweeter than sugar. They are excitotoxins and stimulate the area of the brain that creates a desire for more. These include aspartame, sucralose, saccharin and acesulfame K. Significant amounts of research indicate harmful side effects, including hypertension, cancer-causing compounds and birth defects.

Dairy

Dairy is a modern cultural adaptation and isn't required after weaning; hence most adults no longer produce enough of the enzyme lactase to break down the lactose in the milk, meaning they are lactose intolerant to some degree. As such, dairy isn't an optimal food source for older children or adults. It's estimated that up to 75% of adults worldwide have lost the ability to process lactose since childhood. This ranges from 5% in northern Europe to 70% for southern Europe to 90% or more in some African and Asian countries. The issues are not just related to the carbohydrates in the milk (lactose) but also to the milk proteins (such as casein) and the hormones found in cow's milk (such as bovine insulin, which, research states, is a possible cause of type 1 diabetes in children). Betacellulin, a protein growth factor, has potential links to cancer and type 2 diabetes.

The only reason we currently drink cow's milk is that it has been deemed to be "natural" in modern society. There are no nutrients in milk that cannot be obtained from fresh meat, fish, fruit or vegetables. We should use these foods as the source of those nutrients.

Paleo Nutrition Primer

A balanced diet requires adequate water intake alongside food taken from five nutrient groups. Carbohydrates, proteins and fats are macronutrients used by the body for structure, function and fuel. Vitamins and minerals are micronutrients required in smaller amounts to unlock the energy contained in macronutrients. Ultimately, the quality of food within the diet and chemical composition of that food will have a profound effect on our function, structure and health.

Carbohydrates

"Carbohydrate" is a term used to mean sugars, starches and dietary fiber composed of carbon, hydrogen and oxygen molecules known as saccharides. Carbohydrates are described as simple (like glucose) or complex (like starches such as sweet potatoes). Refined and unrefined carbohydrates are terms that relate to the level of processing involved.

Carbohydrates mostly come from plant-based foods. They're typical sources of dietary fiber, prebiotics and essential nutrients that are crucial for gastrointestinal health. The digestive process breaks down carbohydrates into glucose, which is the form of sugar transported and used by the body. This glucose is used immediately as energy, stored as glycogen in the liver or stored as fat (adipose tissue).

Modern convenience means we often substitute basic fruits and vegetables with cereal grains, sugar and dairy as our primary forms of carbohydrate due to low cost, ease of preparation and extended shelf-life. We can pour cereal grains fortified with vitamins out of a box and simply add milk and sugar; it's far easier than washing, cutting, and preparing fresh vegetables for cooking. Indeed, fruits and vegetables are often overlooked when individuals consider carbohydrate intake, but historically as hunter-gatherers these were our main source of carbohydrates.

Protein

Proteins are composed of smaller building blocks called amino acids. There are several types of proteins used within the body. It isn't just about muscle. Structural proteins form and provide structure to the body, such as collagen in skin, keratin in the nails and elastin in connective tissue. Transport proteins such as hemoglobin in red blood cells are responsible for transporting oxygen around the body. Hormones like insulin are proteins, as are enzymes such as protease and amylase. Dietary proteins are broken down in the stomach and metabolized by the liver. The amino acids are transported by the blood where needed.

Fats

Fats are evil, right? Well, the word strikes fear in many of us. However, fats are a family of compounds called lipids that are essential for our health and are an essential component of our diet. The role of dietary fats is open to considerable debate, but the role that fats play throughout human physiology should not be underestimated.

Fats:

- are part of the structural components of the membrane in every cell in the body;
- constitute the majority of the brain (around 60%), central nervous system and spinal cord;
- maintain the health of blood vessels;
- are involved in the process of making steroid hormones such as testosterone;
- aid in the regulation of enzymes;
- provide insulation through adipose tissue just under the skin and store energy there;
- transport, store and utilize the fat-soluble vitamins A, D, E and K;
- are a high-octane fuel source;
- control inflammation.

Low levels of dietary fat have been linked to memory and learning deficiencies, infertility, increased risk of depression and age-related conditions such as Parkinson's, Alzheimer's and arthritis.

There are three types of fats: saturated, monounsaturated and polyunsaturated. Saturated fats from foods such as eggs and meats are seen as the bad guys. Monounsaturated fats are found in sources such as avocados and olives; polyunsaturated fats from fish, nuts and seeds like sunflower and chia are seen as the good guys. Let's look at saturated fats.

Two now-discredited research papers initiated the idea that cholesterol and saturated fat were linked to heart disease. This concern about fat and cholesterol has been part of our psyche for the last 40 to 50 years. This fat aversion has led us to eat larger proportions of carbohydrates. The first paper, from 1950, revealed that rabbits who are fed a high-cholesterol diet end up with clogged arteries; however, no account was taken of the fact that herbivores were not designed to eat animal fat, which was just as likely an explanation.

The second study published in 1953 by Ancel Keys established a link between saturated fat and heart disease. He discovered that incidences of heart disease in seven countries correlated with levels of fat consumption, starting with Japan, with the lowest levels of fat consumption, through to the U.S., with the highest levels of fat consumption and correspondingly high levels of heart disease. This all sounds impressive until you realize Keyes ignored data from 16 countries that didn't fit his lipid hypothesis, such as, for example, the French and Inuit people, who consumed large quantities of fat and rarely suffered from heart disease.

In the 1970s and 1980s manufacturers began to produce low-fat, no-cholesterol foods, with governments and health institutions continuing to advise consumers of the supposed benefits. Western diets changed radically on that basis. Hydrogenated vegetable fats (industrialized trans fats) such as those in margarine replaced saturated animal fats found in butter. These unnatural trans fats have been found to be highly toxic and are linked to the development of atheroma, a fatty material that builds up within our artery walls, increased abdominal fat and chronic inflammation. Sugars were used as substitutes for fats in low-fat products such as yogurt and cookies, or fats were eliminated entirely, removing even more of the nutrients in the process.

Since Western countries began consuming these foods, there has been an inexorable increase in heart disease. It's now becoming recognized that there are several culprits behind the rise in cardiovascular disease, including hyperinsulinemia (excess levels of insulin), hypertension, inactivity, smoking, drinking, obesity and chronic inflammation.

Essential Fatty Acids

Essential fatty acids (EFAs) are polyunsaturated fats that are essential to the diet since the body is unable to produce these by itself. They help regulate metabolism and prostaglandin (inflammation) activity within the cells. Because this occurs at the cellular level, the effects of prostaglandin and deficiencies in these EFAs can lead to ill health. The two main categories we'll discuss are omega-3 and omega-6 fatty acids. To promote good health, these fatty acids should be eaten in the required amounts and ratio.

Both types of fatty acid are essential, but there's one key difference: omega-6s (like sunflower oil, pumpkin seeds and sesame seeds) are pro-inflammatory and omega-3s (found in oily fish like salmon, walnuts, naturally raised chicken eggs and grass-fed meat) are anti-inflammatory. Maintaining the correct balance of omega-3 and omega-6 fatty acids is vital to human health. Our ancestor's Paleolithic diet provided a ratio of 1:1 while the modern Western diet is closer to 1:16 (omega-3 to omega-6). Studies have shown that excessive amounts of omega-6, or an exceptionally high ratio to omega-3 typical in Western Pattern Diets, promotes inflammation and can contribute to the development of lifestyle diseases such as cardiovascular disease, cancer and autoimmune diseases. Studies suggest the ideal ratio of omega-6 to omega-3 to be between 2:1 and 1:1, similar to the profile above.

In terms of dietary choices, omega-3 fatty acids found in oily fish have been shown to reduce the tendency of blood to clot, lower triglyceride levels and raise HDL (good) cholesterol, which mitigate against risk factors associated with heart disease.

What about Hormones?

Ever wonder why bodies still get fat even when we consume fat-free foods? Hormones play a role in this. Hormones are like messengers in your body that give orders to your cells to do particular things. Let's say you eat a bag of candy, a zero-fat food. Once digested, these carbohydrates are quickly released into the bloodstream as glucose. This blood glucose has to be dealt with, as high concentrations are dangerous. When your body detects the glucose, it releases the hormone insulin to indicate that glucose should be stored as glycogen in muscle and liver cells; any excess turns into fat.

Insulin sensitivity describes how sensitive the body is to the effects of insulin. If sensitivity is low, the body will compensate by producing more insulin. Many people live with high levels of circulating insulin (hyperinsulinemia) due to the high levels of refined and processed carbohydrates in the modern diet. In the presence of insulin, fat cells will not be used for energy. Hyperinsulinemia and abnormally low insulin sensitivity over a prolonged period lead to an inability to regulate normal blood glucose levels and insulin resistance. This is associated with obesity, diabetes, high blood pressure, heart disease, osteoporosis and cancer.

It's crucial to note the body's glucose metabolism is a continuous cycle of glucose, insulin and glucagon. *Glucagon*, a partner hormone to insulin, helps to maintain insulin sensitivity and is important in maintaining lean body mass by releasing energy from fat storage when required. A high-carbohydrate, low-protein diet can lead to too much insulin without adequate glucagon.

Cortisol, the "stress hormone," increases the level of blood sugars and insulin production, breaks down the body's protein and leads to an increase in fat storage, especially around the middle.

Ever wonder why, when overweight, you can still eat very little and struggle to lose weight? *Leptin*, the "satiety hormone" secreted by fat tissue, influences metabolic rate and body fat storage. Leptin signals to the brain how much body fat is stored. If there's enough fat in storage, metabolism increases. If there isn't enough body fat, metabolism slows. In overweight and obese individuals, this signaling mechanism fails. Excess body fat produces too much leptin and the brain cannot regulate metabolism effectively. Termed "leptin resistance," this continuously impedes metabolism and results in more body fat storage. *Ghrelin*, referred to as the "hunger hormone," originates in the stomach and is a counterpart to the leptin. Ghrelin levels increase when the body is hungry and decrease after meals. High levels stimulate appetite, particularly for refined high-carbohydrate foods. There are other chemicals such as Neuropeptide Y which is the key on/off switch for hunger in the brain. This must be switched off for the brain to register satisfaction.

The science behind these appetite hormones isn't yet fully understood, but one thing is abundantly clear: Managing hormone imbalances through diet, exercise, sleep, stress management and avoiding excess abdominal fat will contribute to better health and assist us with understanding that just moving more and eating less isn't necessarily enough.

Managing Hypertension with a Paleo Lifestyle

There are a series of medications available to counter high blood pressure; however, with any medications there are side effects, and usually a cocktail of meds is required to reduce blood pressure. There are healthier alternatives available, one of which is adopting a Paleo lifestyle.

Research has shown that simple lifestyle changes in terms of nutrition and exercise can help to reduce blood pressure. A Paleolithic lifestyle will assist this by:

- reducing salt by avoiding processed, convenience and artificial foods
- avoiding breakfast cereals, which usually contain high levels of salt
- increasing the intake of seasonal fresh vegetables and fruits
- introducing more exposure to so-called functional foods that contain properties that help to reduce blood pressure, such as watermelon, garlic, blueberries and walnuts
- reducing the likelihood of being overweight or having higher than healthy levels of fat, which also contributes to high blood pressure
- minimizing toxins such as coffee and alcohol
- increasing consumption of omega-3 essential fatty acids
- increasing potassium levels found in Paleo staple foods such as fish, nuts, vegetables and eggs, which combat the negative effects of sodium
- increasing activity levels, which has been proven to reduce blood pressure

Fat Loss vs. Weight Loss

Conventional advice teaches that if you burn more calories than you consume, you'll lose weight, and most weight-loss programs work on that basis. But it's becoming increasingly obvious that this formula doesn't always work. If you significantly overeat, then it doesn't matter what you eat—you'll put on weight. However, there are also some people who don't overeat, and yet they, too, have issues managing a healthy body composition. There are also those who exercise excessively and have trouble maintaining a healthy body fat percentage.

A calorie isn't just a calorie. Calorie intake vs. calorie expenditure can't be ignored, but it isn't the only factor when we're talking about managing body composition. Other considerations are the role of hormones like insulin, as well as the crucial differences between fat loss and weight loss, which can be confusing.

Weight loss is the net loss of body weight, for example, a decrease from 150 pounds to 145 pounds. Fat loss is a reduction in overall body fat as a percentage of total body composition; this is factored as a percentage reduction. For example, a loss of 5% total body fat from 25% to 20%.

Here are a few reasons why weight loss usually fails or is the wrong approach to maintaining a truly healthy body: If you're dehydrated, you can appear to lose a few pounds of weight easily. Water loss will directly lead to weight loss. In fact, most people can lose over a pound of "weight" while they're sleeping through water vapor loss while breathing and sweating. The scales may present a result you're happier with, but once you drink to replace "lost" fluids, the pound you lost returns.

You can also restrict calories with a calorie-controlled or crash diet to lose weight. These can be successful in the short term but are unhealthy; in severe cases they can lead to malnutrition (robbing the body of essential nutrients), and can cause the yo-yo diet effect whereby you constantly gain and lose weight for lengthy periods—a vicious cycle of success and failure.

You can lose weight by losing precious lean muscle mass and bone density while increasing the percentage of body fat. In short, maintaining a healthy body fat percentage is more beneficial than staying at an arbitrary "ideal" weight.

Two individuals could be exactly the same weight and height but have different levels of body fat. A 130-pound woman with 35% body fat (clinically obese) will look, feel, and perform differently from a woman who is 130 pounds with 18% body fat (lean and athletic).

Appearances can be deceiving. Evidence suggests the location of your fat has more of a bearing on health than how much fat you have. You could be fat on the inside and appear to be thin outside. A relatively low body weight with a high body fat percentage is known as TOFI (Thin Outside Fat Inside), otherwise termed "skinny fat." This isn't an oxymoron.

The fat we tend to associate with overweight people is subcutaneous fat, the fat just below the surface of the skin. However, millions of people have a fat problem that doesn't put fat on the thighs or the arms. There's fat that's hidden deep inside the body which can be very dangerous. Hidden, internal fat is called visceral fat. Most of this visceral fat surrounds the vital organs such as the liver and kidneys. Visceral fat in itself isn't harmful, but an excess of it is. This fat differs from subcutaneous fat; it's metabolically active and affects other organs quite easily. In one of its most dangerous forms, it can lead to excess epicardial fat, which surrounds the heart.

People who have too much weight around their abdomen, often called an apple shape, have a greater risk of developing heart disease and type 2 diabetes through insulin resistance than those who are pear shaped and carry the weight around the hips. Why is this? Visceral fat releases chemicals that can damage arteries around the heart, leading to heart disease; it also contains chemicals that can increase the likelihood of cancer. With proximity to the liver, visceral fat can affect the liver's ability to clear insulin from the blood, leading to type 2 diabetes.

However, there's some good news: Visceral fat is metabolically active, which means it's some of the first fat that's lost when undertaking a Paleo fitness regime.

Description	Women (body fat %)	Men (body fat %)
Essential Fat	10–13	2–6
Athletic	14–20	7–13
Average	21–24	14–17
Above Average	25–30	18–25
Overfat	31–34	26–30
Obese	35–39	31–35
Morbidly Obese	> 40	> 36

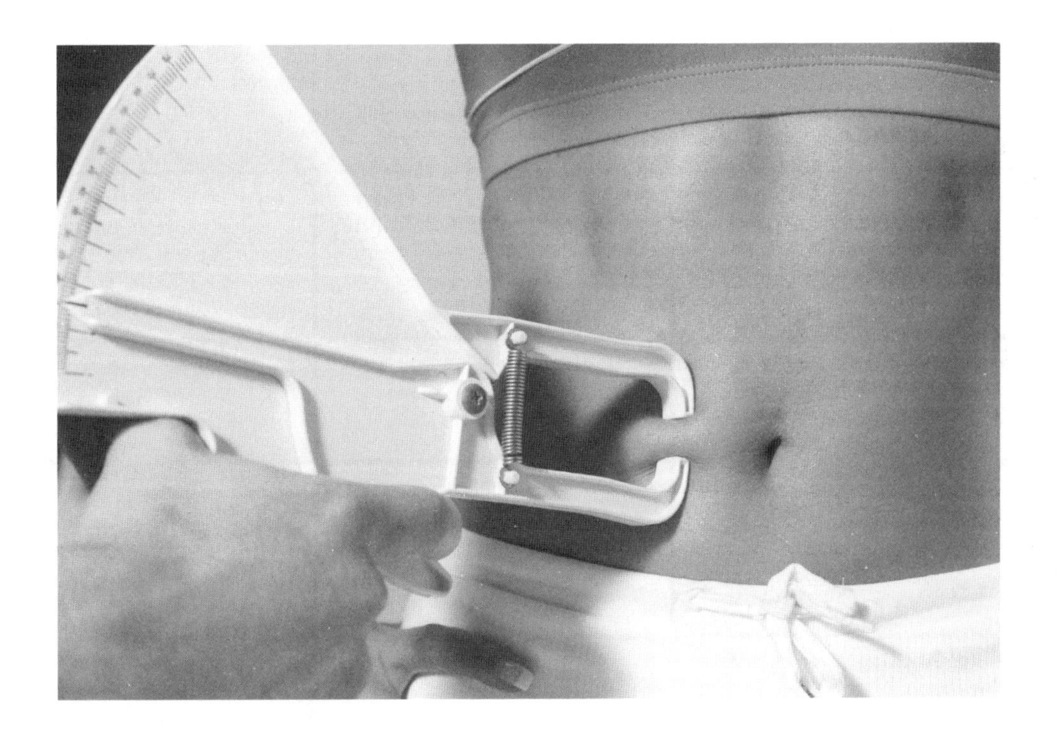

2-WEEK PALEO MEAL PLAN

Week 1			
	Breakfast	Lunch	Dinner
Mon	3 or more hard-boiled eggs and Coconut Surprise "Cereal" (page 157)	Tuna & Avocado Lettuce Wraps (page 157) accompanied by additional cut-up veggies	Salad topped with walnuts, walnut oil and lime juice dressing, and a generous portion of grilled chicken served with a side of sautéed yellow squash, zucchini and red peppers
Tue	Steak and eggs with a side of roasted veggies	6–7 oz. baked white fish with steamed kale and butternut squash	Spicy Chicken Wings (page 145) and a large salad
Wed	Thinly sliced turkey breast with a side of honeydew melon topped with walnuts and a squeeze of fresh lemon juice	Mixed greens salad with grilled sardines and a dressing of avocado oil, thyme, black cracked pepper and lemon juice	Portobello Buffalo Burgers (without bun) (page 155) with Swoon-Worthy Sweet Potatoes (page 145)
Thu	"Pickled" herring and red onions marinated in lemon juice, horseradish, dill allspice, garlic, black peppercorns, a bay leaf and fresh dill, served with a bowl of blueberries and coconut slices and a cup of herbal tea	Salad of shaved fennel, hard-boiled eggs and red radishes with a side of sautéed mushrooms	Sliced roasted turkey and Cauliflower Mash (page 146)
Fri	Half an avocado with a pan-sautéed egg in the middle seasoned with black pepper and paprika	Beef hamburger (without bun) wrapped in lettuce leaves and topped with grilled onions and mushrooms	Leg of lamb and steamed broccoli plus Saffron-Infused Coconut Bars with Toasted Almonds & Pistachios for dessert (page 158)
Sat	Handful of mixed nuts, Granny Smith apple and a cup of Orange Spice Tea (page 160)	Beef and broccoli with a side of peppered mashed yams drizzled with walnut oil	Caribbean Fish Stew (page 144)
Sun	2 eggs "in a basket," using red bell pepper rings instead of bread: slice a bell pepper into thick rings, place in hot pan and crack an egg in the middle	Orange bell peppers stuffed with ground beef, onions and jalapeño pepper	Jamaican Jerk Chicken with Grilled Green Plantains (page 150)

Week 2

	Breakfast	Lunch	Dinner
Mon	Wild Salmon in a Savory Lemon-Dill Sauce (page 156) served with a side salad of sliced cucumbers, shallots, avocados and red bell peppers marinated in avocado oil and lemon juice	Orange roughy broiled in coconut oil and lime juice served with a side of oven-roasted acorn squash with pecans, cinnamon and a pinch of nutmeg	(Chicken) liver and onions stir-fried in avocado oil served with a side of sautéed broccoli and cauliflower
Tue	Scrambled eggs with mushrooms, scallions, and red and green bell peppers	Shirazi Salad (page 147) topped with grilled chicken or beef	Mushroom Pepper Steak (page 152) and oven-roasted sweet potatoes
Wed	Handful of unsalted pistachios plus a bowl of watermelon topped with coconut milk and garnished with fresh mint leaves	Steamed rockfish with a side of sautéed carrots	Spaghetti Squash with Tomato Sauce & Spicy Meatballs (page 148)
Thu	Grilled mackerel marinated in chili, ginger, lime and coconut milk and served with a side of puréed pumpkin mixed with coconut oil	Spinach salad with grilled steak, tomato, hard-boiled egg, avocado and red onion	Pan-Grilled Baby Lamb Chops with Fresh Herbs (page 151) and a Paleo Virgin Mary (page 159)
Fri	Cantaloupe topped with pecans served with a glass of lemon water	Baked turkey breast with rosemary and avocado oil served with a side of sautéed spinach, garlic and Swiss chard	Grilled salmon steak on a bed of asparagus served with oven-baked yams topped with melted coconut oil
Sat	3 poached eggs, cut-up raw vegetables and Iced Coconut Chai (page 159)	Roasted game (or Cornish) hen with a side of grilled eggplant, zucchini and tomatoes	T'ibs We't (Ethiopian Beef Stir-Fry) (page 153) served with a heaping side of sautéed beet greens and garlic tossed in walnut oil
Sun	Roasted pheasant (or chicken) with garlic, fresh rosemary and sage, and mushrooms served with steamed cabbage and a side of apple slices and walnuts sautéed in coconut oil and seasoned with cinnamon	Sweet potato and garlic mash topped with macadamia nuts and seasoned with paprika, rosemary and black pepper	Monkfish in Veracruz Sauce (page 154) and No-Bake Coconut-Hazelnut Bonbons (page 158) for dessert

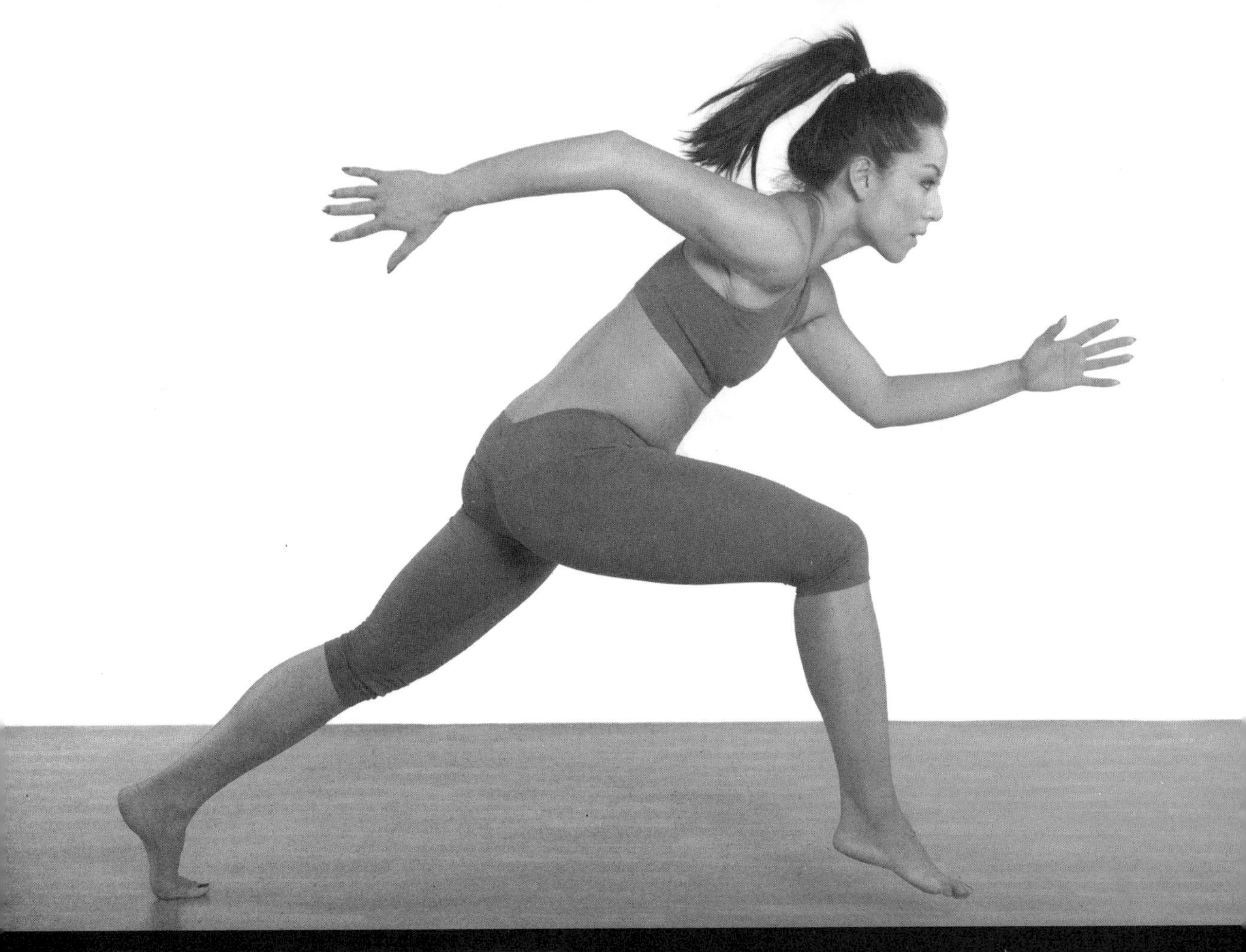

PART III: PALEO WORKOUTS

WHAT IS FITNESS?

At a recent family event, I observed my 60-year-old cousin, and he seemed far younger than his years. There was something about him that had nothing to do with looks or having a young mentality or a surgeon's knife. It was how he moved! His posture, grace, energy and confidence of movement make him appear far younger than his years. His secret? He puts it down to a daily regime of exercise, eating good food, walking, not drinking or smoking and avoiding stress.

One thing is for certain: Our genetic make-up was designed to move, with periods of vigorous daily activity.

Movement

> *Lack of activity destroys the good condition of every human being, while movement and methodical physical exercise save it and preserve it.* —Plato

With the pace of technological innovation in the last century, movement and physical exertion have become increasingly optional. Today we can experience exercise as a hobby rather than deem it an essential part of life. Our ancient ancestors chased prey as hunter-gatherers, walked for miles gathering food and did whatever they could to avoid predators. Several hundred years ago, we were involved extensively with manual labor on farms and factories. We spent more time walking, did housework without the aid of labor-saving devices and spent no time watching TV or playing video games. The proliferation of cars, the decline of agricultural and industrial labor and the abundance of gadgets have all reduced the likelihood of moving, which is evident with the number of adults and children who are now overweight and obese exceeding 1 billion people globally. Those even within normal weight ranges suffer from ailments brought on by being sedentary.

Just like food affects every cell in the body, no organ in the body is unaffected by movement or a lack of it.

Back to Basics

Man's modern environment may have changed dramatically but we can still benefit from moving today as nature intended. We need to be reintroduced to the basic movement patterns that got us here rather than focus on the highly skilled forms of activity that are typical of modern exercise. Instead of seeking out punishing workouts that will get our bodies into shape, we should also focus on general movement that will give us joy and pleasure. A step in the right direction is to enjoy what we can do functionally and practically when fit rather than hating what we have to do to get fit.

PRIMALity

I use the acronym PRIMALity to define the principles of Paleo fitness.

PRACTICAL & PLAYFUL MOVEMENT—Movement that invigorates, is imaginative, is spontaneous, inherently motivates and provides its own reward. We should seek to reclaim the enjoyment of movement that we experienced as children. Beyond function, train for life's challenges, not just for the confines of the gym environment. Don't just work out—play out.

RESTORATIVE MOVEMENT—Movements that regenerate, reinvigorate and restore your body to its natural state of wellness and well-being. This can be done through moves such as performing a squat correctly, comfortably and easily, or lifting a weight with good form for safety.

INSTINCTIVE MOVEMENT—Movement patterns that are universal and which our ancestors did naturally without the rigidity or limitations of modern exercise conventions. These patterns include walking, running, pushing, pulling, jumping, dancing, squatting, balancing, lifting, carrying and so on.

MINDFUL MOVEMENT—Movement in which the mind and body are fully engaged in activity. Focus your mind's attention on your own body, thoughts, emotions and the environment around you. Become curious about your experience.

ADAPTIVE MOVEMENT—The ability to shift among challenges, intensity and disciplines. This adaptability allows your body to be fit and ready for both known and unknown challenges. Performing tasks efficiently, effectively or both.

LIFE-ENHANCING MOVEMENT—Train for the way you want to live. Train for life. Train for longevity.

INTEGRATIVE MOVEMENT—Focus on full-body movement, not muscles. Don't work out to isolate certain muscles, but perform compound, multi-joint exercises that rely on the actions of several muscle groups to move two or more joints through a range of motion.

TACTICAL MOVEMENT—Be opportunistic about movement. Take advantage of opportunities to move whenever possible.

YOUTHFUL MOVEMENT—Movement that exhibits vitality, creativity and passion.

Paleo Fitness Is Versatile Fitness

When we think of fitness, we may conjure up the image of working out in the gym, or maybe playing sports or other outdoor pursuits. We may categorize it into resistance and cardio workouts or break it down further into strength, speed and stamina.

Years ago I came across a list of 10 components of fitness from Dynamax (and adopted by CrossFit). It was the best I had come across: cardiovascular endurance, stamina, strength, flexibility, power, speed, coordination, agility, balance and accuracy. Over the years, I have expanded this list to incorporate 25 attributes that I believe cover all-around fitness.

1. **ACCURACY**—The ability to control movement with precision

2. **AGILITY**—The ability to change the body's position quickly in a controlled fashion

3. **BALANCE**—The ability to control the body's stability while moving or stationary regardless of its base of support

4. **BODY COMPOSITION**—The ability to maintain the optimal ratio of body fat to lean muscle mass

5. **CARDIOVASCULAR ENDURANCE**—The body's ability to gather, process and deliver oxygen

The S.A.I.D Principle and G.P.P.

The S.A.I.D. (Specific Adaptation to Imposed Demands) principle is the base for most athletic training. This is what we do to develop a skill and capability, through much repetition. We adapt to the demands placed on the body on a regular basis. In other words, you get what you train for, and you become what you train.

The more we specialize the more we'll adapt to that stimulus. If I spent all my workout time doing long distances on a bike, the more my body and mind will adapt to cycling—not only in the positive (improving my cardiovascular capacity, slow-twitch muscle fiber capability, endurance capability, lower leg strength and so on) but also in the negative (poor upper body posture, relatively poor upper body strength, increased likelihood of injury, etc.). The same is true of repetitive movements and postures outside of the gym. For example, spending all your time at a desk might result in overly rounded shoulders. We become what we do.

Like our ancestors, we were designed to be multi-disciplined, multi-skilled and multi-faceted, and our training should reflect this. We want to generalize, not specialize.

Unpredictability improves one's capability, and we need constant challenge in order to adapt. Sometimes our workouts should be unstructured, unplanned, irregular, and unorthodox. Sometimes we should change based on what we can take advantage of at the time or to deal with a situation that's unexpected. For example, a pull-up on the bar in the gym doesn't mean you can perform a pull-up on a tree branch that requires a wider and uneven grip.

Although we can spend our time focusing on movement patterns required for sport-specific training, as human beings we thrive on a wider repertoire of movements not only in terms of physicality but also enjoyment. G.P.P. (General Physical Preparedness) is a technique used by sport coaches to cover all fitness bases, improvements in flexibility, strength, cardiovascular fitness, speed and endurance.

6. **COORDINATION**—The ability to combine several distinct movements into one integrated move
7. **EFFICIENCY**—The ability to perform movement with minimal exertion
8. **EXTEROCEPTION**—The ability to respond to stimuli outside the body
9. **FLEXIBILITY**—Optimal range of movement at the joints
10. **FLOW**—The mental state of being entirely focused on the task at hand
11. **FUNCTION**—The ability to perform whatever activity is required
12. **MINDFULNESS**—The ability to be aware, careful and thoughtful about movement
13. **MOBILITY**—The ability to move freely and easily
14. **MUSCULAR ENDURANCE**—The ability of muscles to maintain force production over time
15. **POSTURE**—The ability to maintain the correct alignment and position of limbs while moving or stationary
16. **POWER**—The ability to exert maximum strength explosively over a given distance
17. **PROPRIOCEPTION**—The internal awareness of the body's position in relation to its environment
18. **RECOVERY TIME**—The ability for the body to return to its preactivity state after exercise
19. **RESPONSE TIME**—The ability to react quickly (and appropriately) to external stimuli
20. **SKILL**—The ability to develop gross and fine motor skills to refine technique

21. SPEED—The ability to move as quickly as possible over a given distance

22. STAMINA—The body's ability to process, store and utilize energy for a sustained work effort

23. STRENGTH—The ability to exert a force against resistance using your own body weight or external objects

24. STRENGTH ENDURANCE—The ability to apply force against resistance for a sustained period

25. SUSTENANCE—The ability to provide the body with the nutrients required for good health, repair and optimal performance

In a nutshell, Paleo fitness is the ability to perform daily, recreational and extraordinary physical tasks efficiently and/or effectively.

Functional Paleo Training

There is no better training ground than the real world. Studies, common sense and my own personal experience and those of my clients all reveal that those who exercise for health-related reasons as opposed to appearance-related reasons maintain an exercise program for the long term. Focus on health.

The human body should be able to switch between fast, powerful movement and slow, controlled movement. Fast movements are required to adequately stress the nervous system, slow and isometric movements to support the muscle and soft tissue structures. This mimics real-life physical demands and is also beneficial for sports-specific training for activities such as rugby, football and MMA. Every move we cover in *Paleo Fitness* is a full-body exercise, and you should focus on movement, not muscles. Through movements we learned as children we can help our bodies improve flexibility, improve recovery time, prevent injury, and increase stamina and strength. We'll also do calisthenics and strength work to combat the effects of aging.

Make Your Daily Activity Physical Activity

In the beginner's mind there are many possibilities, in the expert's mind there are few. —Shunryu Suzuki

Don't feel that exercise needs to be conducted at a certain time or place. Simply increase the amount of low-intensity daily activity you engage in. Avoid segregating or isolating movement in your day-to-day life. If you consider exercise a hobby, then you will fit it in after all the other priorities. Instead, make physical activity something you do all the time by generally avoiding sedentary options. It doesn't mean you have to devote all your time to movement. Just look for ways to increase activity: Take the stairs rather than the elevator, run for the bus, walk to the local grocery, stand up when talking on the phone, take activity breaks away from sitting down all day at the office. This will ensure a more enriching and active life. It's as easy as getting out and about.

Recent studies about sedentary lifestyles have given rise to a new field of medical research called inactivity physiology, which explores the effects of an ever-increasing amount of our lives being tied to sitting down. Some researchers are even calling this "sitting disease."

Walking as much as our ancestors did is often overlooked today. Research has shown that walking:

- reduces the risk of lifestyle diseases such as coronary heart disease, stroke and type 2 diabetes;

- reduces risk of hypertension (high blood pressure);
- reduces high cholesterol;
- helps to prevent osteoporosis by increasing bone density;
- enhances mental well-being (less prone to depression and anxiety);
- relieves osteoarthritis;
- reduces mortality rates for both younger and older adults;
- reduces the risk of senile dementia.

The ideal cumulative weekly distance was found to be between 6 and 9 miles a week, with no significant improvement walking any farther.

Maximize the Benefits of Exercise—Connect with Nature

Take the opportunity to go outside to train. Research tells us the profound impact that fresh air, grass, trees and colors in the natural environment have on mental health and physical well-being. A study at the University of Queensland, Australia, found that those who exercised outdoors on a regular basis had higher levels of serotonin, a hormone that regulates mood, than those who exercised mainly indoors. They also had higher levels of endorphins, the post-exercise rush that occurs after exercise.

Science even has a term for this: biophilia. It literally means "love of life" and refers to the love we have for the natural world. We don't need science to confirm that being outdoors is good for us; most of us feel this instinctively. Evidence for biophilia demonstrates that exposure to and interaction with nature can have a profound effect on mental performance, self-awareness, vitality, and appreciation of our environment and others.

Being outside more is also associated with higher levels of vitamin D because of additional sun exposure. This has significant health benefits, including boosting the immune system, improving heart health, improving calcium absorption and bone health and preventing cancer.

Interval Training

Everything we do is based on intervals: changes of tempo, speed and intensity. Watch children play. It's rare that they do the same movement continuously; that would be boring. What usually happens is they work in bursts of super-charged activity, then walk around to recover, then work at different levels of intensity playing something else. Take a game as easy as tag. All energy systems are involved: high-speed sprints, deceleration, pivoting, periods of recovery, slow running, agility, balance and coordination. Instead of running in a straight line and predicting what will happen when, everything is tactical.

It's no wonder that scientists have identified training in this fashion as the best way to boost metabolism and burn fat. There's a significant amount of evidence that short bursts of high-intensity anaerobic training such as sprinting is more effective for fat-loss than continuous low-intensity aerobic exercise, such as jogging. This is the case even though overall total calories burned may be higher in the aerobic exercise, and exercise time may be significantly lower for the anaerobic exercise—go figure! High-intensity exercise is associated with higher levels of HDL (good) cholesterol, accounting for a decreased risk of heart disease.

GETTING STARTED WITH PALEO FITNESS

Having access to knowledge about healthy foods and exercise isn't enough to make change happen. Fortunately, there's a way to selectively sift through the vast quantities of conflicting food advice, opinion and marketing hype and arrive at what you can feel confident about: going back to basics.

The first step before we commence is to have a plan, in this case becoming more mindful about what you eat and improving your knowledge about food, nutrition and movement. We often choose goals that are somewhat vague, such as "I want to lose weight" or "I want to get fitter and healthier." Even with all the positive energy around New Year's resolutions, over 85% of them fail, and usually within a few weeks! So having a strategy for integrating and making positive changes to our lifestyle is advantageous. For example, what does getting fitter and healthier mean? How do we know if we're successful, or at least moving in the right direction?

Be S.M.A.R.T. and Set Goals

S.M.A.R.T is an acronym used in project management for goal setting. It stands for specific, measurable, achievable, relevant and timed, and it works well outside the business world, too. This is a simple method I give my clients to implement lasting change and to ensure it's framed around health gain, rather than just weight loss.

SPECIFIC—Specify exactly what you want from your goal, and be precise here. Think about what you really want, down to the last detail.

MEASURABLE—Can you measure and track your success? It's useful to provide a feedback mechanism that will ensure you can monitor progress.

ACHIEVABLE—Set an objective you can realistically attain. Use whatever resources to determine what this realistic level should be.

RELEVANT—Is this a suitable goal for YOU and you alone? Everyone has unique areas to improve upon.

TIMED—Determine a time frame for this goal. Set regular intervals to record and check progress from start to finish.

What does this mean in terms of applying this to our lifestyle changes? Here's a S.M.A.R.T. goal example:

> *I will lose an average of 2 pounds of body fat per week, decrease my waist size by 2 inches, improve my body fat percentage from 19% to 14% and reduce my high blood pressure by increasing my activity levels, following a Paleo-type diet and getting adequate sleep. I will do this within eight weeks. I will know I'm making progress because I will take weekly measurements.*

Find a quiet place to really think about your goal. Visualize it, write it down and put it somewhere you can see it often. Focus on want you want for yourself, and finish the following sentence:

> *I will [your goal(s)] by [what you'll do to achieve it]. I will do this within/by [enter time frame/end date]. I will*

ensure I'm making progress because [how you'll monitor progress].

Ensure your goal covers health, fitness, mental state (for example, relating to reducing stress levels) and social interaction (for example, "I will do one partner-based session a week with a friend to increase motivation").

Additional ways to increase the likelihood of success:

- Make your goals public and enlist the help of friends and family to encourage and provide support. This is the best thing any of us can do to improve our health and attitude toward it.
- Know that it takes hard work and determination in order to transform your life and conquer the challenges that will make that change happen.
- Set yourself small, measurable sub-tasks (think tiny baby steps that feel good in the moment rather than huge strides) so the larger goal is easier to accomplish.
- Remember that some days will be easy and others will be difficult. Having an off day or week doesn't equate to failure. Just continue on your well-being journey.
- Write your achievements down. Create a checklist and mark these off upon completion.
- Think about several reasons for making this change and focus on these when you lack motivation.
- Once you've set your goal, recognize that wanting it isn't enough—nothing can be accomplished without taking action!

Pictures & Measurements

After your goal-setting exercise, take your "before" picture. As your body composition improves, the changes in how you look and feel occur gradually so you may not notice them from day to day. Comparing your appearance before you start the *Paleo Fitness* program with how you do along the way and after will make your progress obvious. In addition to a head shot, get full-length and profile photos.

Next, record your measurements: weight and body fat percentage (preferably using a body fat scale or calipers). Each week at the same time, record your weight, waist and hip measurements, blood pressure, resting heart rate and body fat percentage. See "Measurements for Health" in the Appendix on page 138 for the best ways to measure each parameter. You should also get a few standard blood tests to check a few key biomarkers of health. Check your progress using the measurements and chart on page 142.

PALEO FITNESS PROGRAMS

Here are three key objectives of the *Paleo Fitness* program:

1. To improve overall health and fitness by striving for uniformity across all 25 fitness components
2. To make activities varied, functional, practical, enjoyable and adaptive
3. To work out, play out, experiment and explore

The aim of the programs in this book is to arrange for fitness activities that cover previously sedentary individuals, weekend warriors and those looking for more challenging workouts based on natural movements. We're all natural athletes. We may differ in terms of ability but not in the baseline requirements of moving. We'll use interval training and circuits to improve the effectiveness of the program. All the exercises follow the same rules:

- The activity must be safe (laws of common sense apply).
- The exercise must be easy to learn but challenging to master.
- The exercise does not require elaborate equipment.
- The exercise trains movement and does not target individual muscles.
- The exercise should help regain the enjoyment of movement.

Paleo Circuits

One day a week of each program will follow this form. Instead of an abrupt stop/start of exercises, we want an uninterrupted flow of movements of constantly varied speed and intensity. String the exercises into one continuous flow of movement, transitioning from one move to the next. This is a natural way to move. Think of this as a slow-paced workout to focus on form and technique with occasional bursts of increased intensity.

Resting during Activity

Rest as required during any of the activities, but instead of just standing hunched over to catch your breath, stand tall and walk. This is known as active recovery. It'll be far easier to breathe and will increase the amount of movement per workout as well as improve the rate of recovery over time. For example, if you're engaging in a crawling motion then rest on all fours in a comfortable position and begin moving again at the first possible opportunity.

Play Out, Don't Just Work Out

Playful movement is that which invigorates: It's imaginative, spontaneous and inherently motivational, and provides its own reward. Make these activities fun as well as challenging. Use your imagination to create scenarios that will make the workouts more interesting. For example, when doing a bear crawl, imagine you're crawling under a low-hanging branch covered in thorns. It sounds like child's play, but engaging the brain in this fashion can actually increase muscle activation and make you work harder. This is one reason athletes often use visualization when training to improve their athletic performance.

Scientific studies demonstrate that visualization brings about quantifiable improvements as well as physiological changes. Research has also shown that using mental imagery for muscle movement can create similar electrical activity as that seen during actual movement. Imagination also helps to increase motivation and allows us to create whatever environment we need to accomplish our goals.

Tabata Intervals

Tabata intervals are a protocol based on 20 seconds of high-intensity work, such as sprinting, followed by 10 seconds of rest for 8 rounds (4 minutes total). The Tabata protocol is a training method that was originally used by the Japanese Olympic speed skating team and is based on the work of scientist Izumi Tabata. The key finding from the research was that a short period—4 minutes—of this high-intensity interval gave the same improvements to the aerobic system (exercise using oxygen) as 60 minutes of moderate-intensity exercise. The other key difference was an increase in the anaerobic system ability (exercise capability at the highest intensity without oxygen). This anaerobic system was not improved at all with moderate-intensity exercise.

The Importance of Warm-Ups

Warm-ups will increase body temperature and heart rate, and stimulate the entire body and its biomechanical functions. They're useful practice for basic movement patterns and help to prepare for more vigorous training. Some rules for warm-ups: Keep warm-ups short and focused—they shouldn't be completely exhausting but neither should they be at a relaxed pace.

- Get out of breath and feel a light sweat.
- Make sure joints are loosened and limbered up.
- Make sure muscles are warm.
- Be mentally and physically prepared for the activity at hand. Make sure the whole body is warming up.

What about Stretching?

There are hundreds of studies about stretching that are pretty much inconclusive. Some studies reveal that static stretches negatively impact exercise performance, while others say that any increases in flexibility are transitory and increase the likelihood of injury. Other research points to a promotion of relaxation, while other studies report that stretches increase tension in the muscles. The stretches that appear to be the most beneficial from research are dynamic stretches (think stretching with movement), but only in terms of not being detrimental rather than offering significant value.

For *Paleo Fitness*, we'll take our cue from nature. Ever seen a cat contract its muscles and yawn? It appears to be just a one-second stretch, but it isn't. Animals don't stretch to become flexible, they pandiculate. A static stretch is usually working on a muscle in isolation to a point of discomfort. Pandiculation is a short, full-body contraction of muscles that work together without discomfort (usually accompanied with a yawn) and then a relaxation of the body.

Animals move frequently to move well. They work with vigorous, daily, full-body movement, a prescription for health, agility, endurance and strength. For humans, moving consistently and naturally will lengthen the muscles and help us regain the range of motion we had as children. You should aim to be agile, supple and childlike in your movements. Pandiculation has been linked to vitality and exuberance in animals. Choose to pandiculate whenever possible.

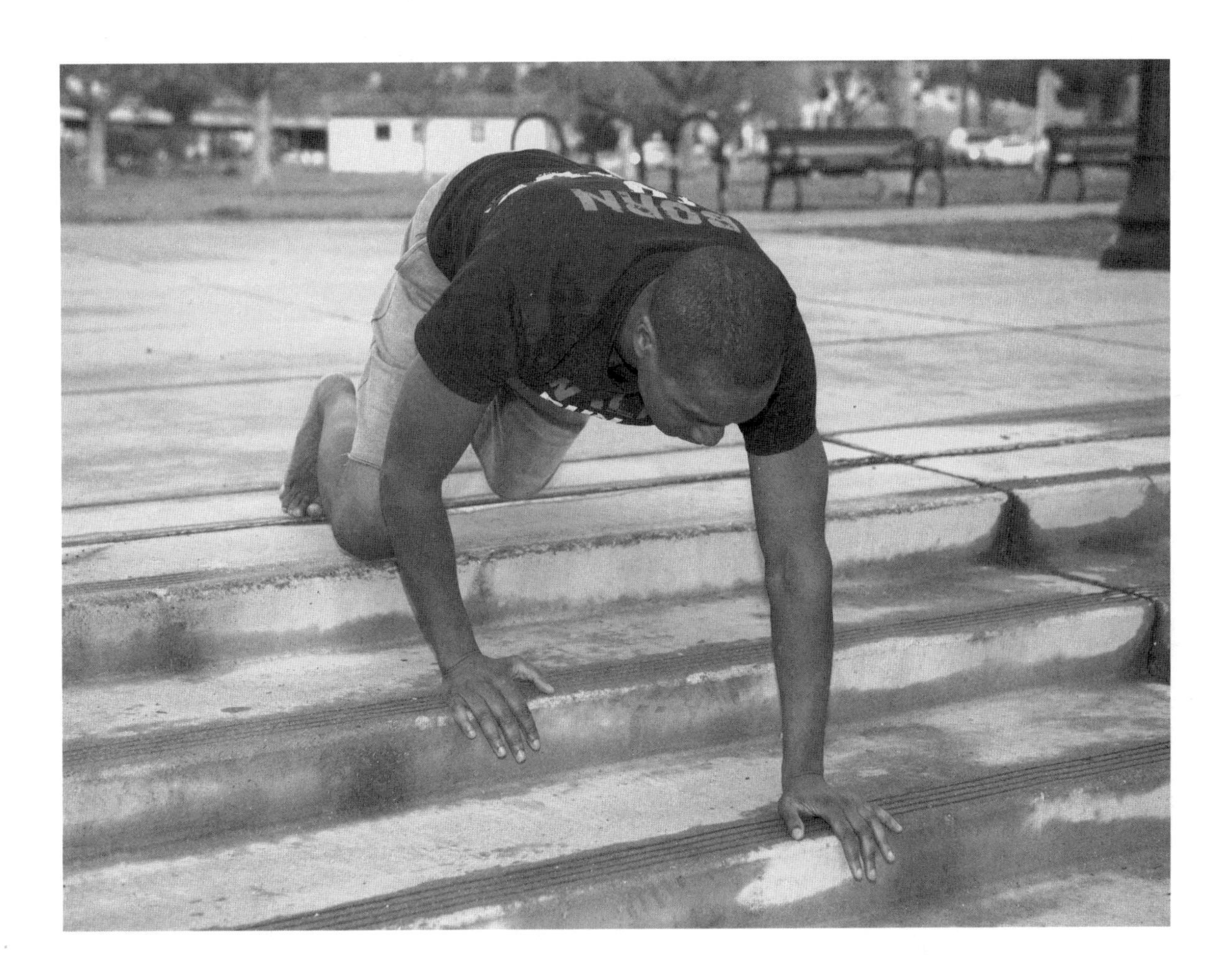

WEEKLY PROGRAMMING

These workout plans will have you exercising up to six days a week. That may sound like a lot, especially if you're just starting a workout routine like this for the first time. But there's built-in flexibility to work around your schedule and days that you're recovering by doing activity such as walking. This is how we'll break down each day:

Monday

Monday is movement technique and focus day. Based on what we call a Paleo circuit, here we focus on technique and play around with differing levels of intensity while working on the flow between exercises. Today is a mandatory day, around 30 minutes of work, plus 5–10 minutes each day required for warm-ups and cool-downs.

Tuesday and Thursday

Tuesday and Thursday are high-intensity Tabata interval days. Here you want to give it everything you have! Aim to make Tuesday mandatory each week. For example, if you're feeling particularly sore or need more time to recover from a previous day's session, you can make Thursday optional. For beginners, this will start as a 4–5 minute workout (including recovery period), leading up to 20 minutes for level 3 participants.

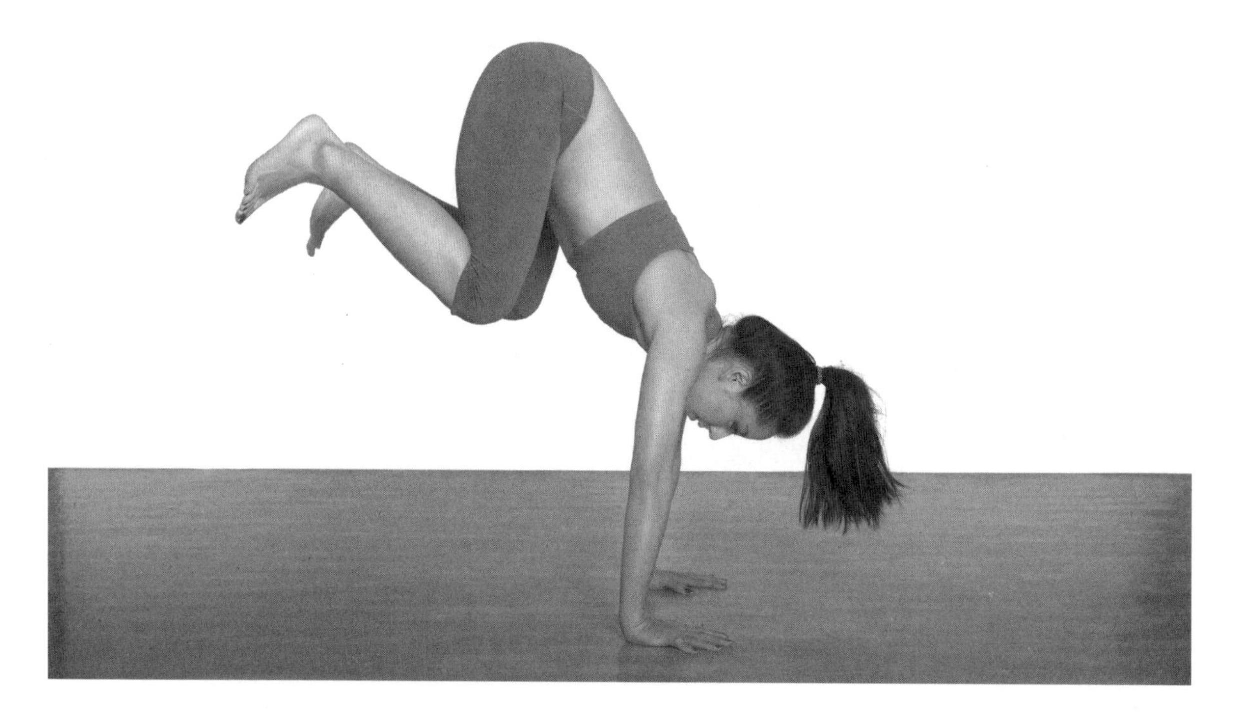

Wednesday

Wednesday is a day to focus on walking. Don't use this as an excuse to do nothing as a day of rest or to do another workout. Take pleasure in breaking the usual routine and go for a walk. This is not a power-walking exercise. Walk at a very leisurely pace.

Friday

Friday is a day of fun. Maybe you can try something you haven't done before, or take an opportunity to play. Try not to engage in a sport or very intense activity. Today is more about stressing the fun element rather than your body. It could be playing tag or catch with the kids, playing frisbee, or learning to Rollerblade.

Saturday

Saturday focuses on some strength training and sprinting work. Like Tabata days, the work is very short but very intense!

Sunday

Sunday is a day of relaxation. If you follow the program as prescribed for the week, then you'll notice there are only three days of intense and vigorous activity, and three days of low-to-moderate activity. And the workouts are so short that the time component also isn't excessive even for those with a busy schedule.

The plan is flexible enough that you can adjust it to fit your schedule. For example, you could make Saturday your day for relaxing instead of Sunday. Or you could replace Thursday's workout with Saturday's if you have no spare time on the weekend. Just make sure you don't have two high-intensity days back-to-back. This won't give you adequate time to recover, you won't be able to work hard enough on the second day to reap maximum benefit or this could lead to injury.

Try to make movement the primary focus. Don't think of it as training anymore. Training is usually working to achieve a goal, a hobby or a set discipline. We want our movement to be completely interwoven into everything that we do. Choose to challenge yourself with movement.

If you feel comfortable being barefoot for most or all of the activities, then feel free to do so. See page 162 for more details on going barefoot.

LEVEL I

Level I: Week 1

Movement Monday	Paleo Circuit		
Exercise	**Distance/Time/Reps**	**Rest**	**Rounds**
Crab Walk p. 96	5 meters		
Duck Walk p. 101	5 meters		
Bear Crawl p. 94	5 meters		
Jumping Pull-Up p. 107	5 reps		
Barefoot Walk Drill p. 70	30 seconds		
Repeat for 30 minutes, rest as required.			

Tabata Tuesday	Tabata protocol (maximum intensity for 20 seconds, rest for 10 seconds)		
Exercise	**Distance/Time/Reps**	**Rest**	**Rounds**
Jump Rope p. 117	20 seconds	10 seconds	2
Walk	30 seconds		
Upper Body Sprint p. 119	20 seconds	10 seconds	2
Walk	30 seconds		
Lunge p. 76	20 seconds	10 seconds	2
Walk	30 seconds		
Get-Up/Stand-Up p. 83	20 seconds	10 seconds	2
Walk	1 minute		
Hunter-Gatherer Squat p. 92	Hold as long as possible		

Walk Wednesday	Walk for 30 minutes. No power walking required. Be slow and mindful.

Tabata Thursday	Tabata protocol (maximum intensity for 20 seconds, rest for 10 seconds)		
Exercise	**Distance/Time/Reps**	**Rest**	**Rounds**
Jumping Pull-Up p. 107	20 seconds	10 seconds	2
Walk	30 seconds		
Standing Push-Up p. 79	20 seconds	10 seconds	2
Walk	30 seconds		
Squat p. 74	20 seconds	10 seconds	2
Walk	30 seconds		
Sprinting in Place p. 120	20 seconds	10 seconds	2
Walk	1 minute		
Inverted Hang p. 111	Hold as long as possible		

Fun Friday	Do something really playful today.

Super Saturday			
Exercise	**Distance/Time/Reps**	**Rest**	**Rounds**
Piggy Back p. 126	20 meters		
Barefoot Walk Drill p. 70	2 minutes		
Crouch to Sprint p. 118	15 seconds		
Barefoot Walk Drill p. 70	2 minutes		
Repeat for 2 rounds total.			

Slow Down Sunday	Relax.

Level I: Week 2

Movement Monday	Paleo Circuit		
Exercise	**Distance/Time/Reps**	**Rest**	**Rounds**
Bunny Hop (on the spot) p. 113	10 reps		
Backward Bear Crawl p. 94	5 meters		
Toddler Climb p. 102	6 reps		
Crab Walk p. 96	5 meters		
Barefoot Walk Drill p. 70	30 seconds		
Repeat for 30 minutes, rest as required.			

Tabata Tuesday	Tabata protocol (maximum intensity for 20 seconds, rest for 10 seconds)		
Exercise	**Distance/Time/Reps**	**Rest**	**Rounds**
Tuck Jump p. 114	20 seconds	10 seconds	2
Walk	30 seconds		
Bear Crawl p. 94	20 seconds	10 seconds	2
Walk	30 seconds		
Prisoner Squat p. 74	20 seconds	10 seconds	2
Walk	30 seconds		
Get-Up/Stand-Up p. 83	20 seconds	10 seconds	2
Walk	1 minute		
Arm Plank p. 90	Hold as long as possible		

Walk Wednesday	Walk for 30 minutes. No power walking required. Be slow and mindful.

Tabata Thursday	Tabata protocol (maximum intensity for 20 seconds, rest for 10 seconds)		
Exercise	**Distance/Time/Reps**	**Rest**	**Rounds**
Jumping Pull-Up p. 107	20 seconds	10 seconds	3
Walk	30 seconds		
Chair Dip p. 81	20 seconds	10 seconds	3
Walk	30 seconds		
Thruster p. 78	20 seconds	10 seconds	3
Walk	30 seconds		
Resisted Arm Press p. 84	20 seconds	10 seconds	3
Walk	1 minute		
Dead Hang p. 104	Hold as long as possible		

Fun Friday	Do something really playful today.

Super Saturday			
Exercise	**Distance/Time/Reps**	**Rest**	**Rounds**
Deadlift p. 129	10 reps	2 minutes	
Crouch to Sprint p. 118	15 seconds	2 minutes	
Repeat for 3 rounds total.			

Slow Down Sunday	Relax.

Level I: Week 3

Movement Monday	Paleo Circuit		
Exercise	**Distance/Time/Reps**	**Rest**	**Rounds**
Kangaroo Jump p. 116	10 meters		
Duck Walk p. 101	10 meters		
Backward Crab Walk p. 96	5 meters		
Forward Bunny Hop p. 113	5 meters	30 seconds	
Repeat for 30 minutes.			

Tabata Tuesday	Tabata protocol (maximum intensity for 20 seconds, rest for 10 seconds)		
Exercise	**Distance/Time/Reps**	**Rest**	**Rounds**
Tuck Jump p. 114	20 seconds	10 seconds	3
Walk	30 seconds		
Toddler Climb p. 102	20 seconds	10 seconds	3
Walk	30 seconds		
Clockwork Lunge p. 77	20 seconds	10 seconds	3
Walk	30 seconds		
Get-Up/Stand-Up p. 83	20 seconds	10 seconds	3
Walk	1 minute		
Hunter-Gatherer Squat p. 92	Hold as long as possible		

Walk Wednesday	Walk for 45 minutes. No power walking required. Be slow and mindful.

Tabata Thursday	Tabata protocol (maximum intensity for 20 seconds, rest for 10 seconds)		
Exercise	Distance/Time/Reps	Rest	Rounds
Standing Push-Up p. 79	20 seconds	10 seconds	3
Walk	30 seconds		
Prisoner Squat p. 74	20 seconds	10 seconds	3
Walk	30 seconds		
Inverted Row p. 112	20 seconds	10 seconds	3
Walk	30 seconds		
Squat Thrust p. 88	20 seconds	10 seconds	3
Walk	1 minute		
Chin-Over p. 105	Hold as long as possible		

Fun Friday	Do something really playful today.

Super Saturday			
Exercise	Distance/Time/Reps	Rest	Rounds
Piggy Back p. 126	10 meters		
Crouch to Sprint p. 118	20 seconds	2 minutes	
Repeat for 4 rounds total.			

Slow Down Sunday	Relax.

Level I: Week 4

Movement Monday	Paleo Circuit		
Exercise	**Distance/Time/Reps**	**Rest**	**Rounds**
Crouch to Sprint p. 118	10 meters		
Crab Walk p. 96	5 meters		
Pull-Up p. 106	1 rep		
Crab Walk p. 96	5 meters		
Backward Bunny Hop p. 113	5 meters		
Pull-Up p. 106	1 rep	30 seconds	
Repeat for 30 minutes, rest as required.			

Tabata Tuesday	Tabata protocol (maximum intensity for 20 seconds, rest for 10 seconds)		
Exercise	**Distance/Time/Reps**	**Rest**	**Rounds**
Squat Jump p. 115	20 seconds	10 seconds	4
Walk	30 seconds		
Upper Body Sprint p. 119	20 seconds	10 seconds	4
Walk	30 seconds		
Jump Rope p. 117	20 seconds	10 seconds	4
Walk	30 seconds		
Crossover Knee p. 87	20 seconds	10 seconds	4
Walk	1 minute		
Hunter-Gatherer Squat p. 92	Hold as long as possible		

Walk Wednesday	Walk for 45 minutes. No power walking required. Be slow and mindful.

Tabata Thursday	Tabata protocol (maximum intensity for 20 seconds, rest for 10 seconds)		
Exercise	Distance/Time/Reps	Rest	Rounds
Jump Pull-Up p. 106	20 seconds	10 seconds	4
Walk	30 seconds		
Chair Dip p. 81	20 seconds	10 seconds	4
Walk	30 seconds		
Prisoner Squat p. 74	20 seconds	10 seconds	4
Walk	30 seconds		
Push-Up p. 79	20 seconds	10 seconds	4
Walk	1 minute		
Dead Hang p. 104	Hold as long as possible		

Fun Friday	Do something really playful today.

Super Saturday			
Exercise	Distance/Time/Reps	Rest	Rounds
Front Squat p. 74	10 reps		
Farmer's Walk	25 meters		
Crouch to Sprint p. 118	15 seconds	2 minutes	
Repeat for 5 rounds total.			

Slow Down Sunday	Relax.

LEVEL II

Level II: Week 1

Movement Monday	Paleo Circuit		
Exercise	**Distance/Time/Reps**	**Rest**	**Rounds**
Kangaroo Jump p. 116	10 meters		
Crab Walk p. 96	15 meters		
Duck Walk p. 101	10 meters		
Cat Walk	15 meters		
Jumping Pull-Up p. 107	10 reps		
Back Extension p. 85	10 reps		
Barefoot Walk Drill p. 70	30 seconds		
Repeat for 30 minutes, rest as required.			

Tabata Tuesday	Tabata protocol (maximum intensity for 20 seconds, rest for 10 seconds)		
Exercise	**Distance/Time/Reps**	**Rest**	**Rounds**
Jump Rope p. 117	20 seconds	10 seconds	4
Walk	30 seconds		
Toddler Climb p. 102	20 seconds	10 seconds	4
Walk	30 seconds		
Walking Lunge p. 76	20 seconds	10 seconds	4
Walk	30 seconds		
Backward Bear Crawl p. 94	20 seconds	10 seconds	4
Walk	1 minute		
Dead Hang p. 104	Hold as long as possible		

Walk Wednesday	Walk for 45 minutes. No power walking required. Be slow and mindful.

Tabata Thursday	Tabata protocol (maximum intensity for 20 seconds, rest for 10 seconds)		
Exercise	**Distance/Time/Reps**	**Rest**	**Rounds**
Jump Pull-Up p. 106	20 seconds	10 seconds	4
Walk	30 seconds		
Waiter's Walk	20 seconds	10 seconds	4
Walk	30 seconds		
Backward Crab Walk p. 96	20 seconds	10 seconds	4
Walk	30 seconds		
Salamander Press-Up p. 98	20 seconds	10 seconds	4
Walk	1 minute		
Hunter-Gatherer Squat p. 92	Hold as long as possible		

Fun Friday	Do something really playful today.

Super Saturday			
Exercise	**Distance/Time/Reps**	**Rest**	**Rounds**
Piggy Back p. 126	40 meters		
Shoulder-to-Shoulder Press p. 132	5 reps		
Barefoot Walk Drill p. 70	1 minute		
Crouch to Sprint p. 118	20 seconds		
Barefoot Walk Drill p. 70	2 minutes		
Repeat for 3 rounds total.			

Slow Down Sunday	Relax.

Level II: Week 2

Movement Monday	Paleo Circuit		
Exercise	**Distance/Time/Reps**	**Rest**	**Rounds**
Bunny Hop p. 113	10 meters		
Backward Bear Crawl p. 94	10 meters		
Tuck Jump p. 114	5 reps		
Toddler Climb p. 102	20 reps		
Backward Crab Walk p. 96	5 meters		
Pull-Up p. 106	3 reps		
Walk	30 seconds		
Repeat for 30 minutes, rest as required.			

Tabata Tuesday	Tabata protocol (maximum intensity for 20 seconds, rest for 10 seconds)		
Exercise	**Distance/Time/Reps**	**Rest**	**Rounds**
Squat Thrust p. 88	20 seconds	10 seconds	4
Walk	30 seconds		
Crossover Knee p. 87	20 seconds	10 seconds	4
Walk	30 seconds		
Tuck Jump p. 114	20 seconds	10 seconds	4
Walk	30 seconds		
Overhead Lunge p. 76	20 seconds	10 seconds	4
Walk	1 minute		
Gorilla Plank p. 90	Hold as long as possible		

Walk Wednesday	Walk for 45 minutes. No power walking required. Be slow and mindful.

Tabata Thursday	Tabata protocol (maximum intensity for 20 seconds, rest for 10 seconds)		
Exercise	**Distance/Time/Reps**	**Rest**	**Rounds**
Jump Pull-Up p. 106	20 seconds	10 seconds	4
Walk	30 seconds		
Chair Dip p. 81	20 seconds	10 seconds	4
Walk	30 seconds		
Squat p. 74	20 seconds	10 seconds	4
Walk	30 seconds		
Resisted Arm Press p. 84	20 seconds	10 seconds	4
Walk	1 minute		
Hunter-Gatherer Squat p. 92	Hold as long as possible		

Fun Friday	Do something really playful today.

Super Saturday			
Exercise	**Distance/Time/Reps**	**Rest**	**Rounds**
Deadlift p. 129	10		
Crouch to Sprint p. 118	20 seconds	3 minutes	
Repeat for 3 rounds total.			

Slow Down Sunday	Relax.

Level II: Week 3

Movement Monday	Paleo Circuit		
Exercise	**Distance/Time/Reps**	**Rest**	**Rounds**
Rabbit Walk p. 99	10 meters		
Duck Walk p. 101	10 meters		
Pull-Up p. 106	4 reps		
Backward Bunny Hop p. 113	5 meters		
Back Extension p. 85	10 reps	30 seconds	
Repeat for 30 minutes, rest as required.			

Tabata Tuesday	Tabata protocol (maximum intensity for 20 seconds, rest for 10 seconds)		
Exercise	**Distance/Time/Reps**	**Rest**	**Rounds**
Burpee p. 89	20 seconds	10 seconds	5
Walk	1 minute		
Upper Body Sprint p. 119	20 seconds	10 seconds	5
Walk	1 minute		
Crab Walk p. 96	20 seconds	10 seconds	5
Walk	1 minute		
Get-Up/Stand-Up p. 83	20 seconds	10 seconds	5
Walk	1 minute		
Gorilla Plank p. 90	Hold as long as possible		

Walk Wednesday	Walk for 45 minutes. No power walking required. Be slow and mindful.

Tabata Thursday

Tabata protocol (maximum intensity for 20 seconds, rest for 10 seconds)

Exercise	Distance/Time/Reps	Rest	Rounds
Push-Up p. 79	20 seconds	10 seconds	5
Walk	1 minute		
Tuck Jump p. 114	20 seconds	10 seconds	5
Walk	1 minute		
Squat p. 74	20 seconds	10 seconds	5
Walk	1 minute		
Toddler Traverse p. 103	20 seconds	10 seconds	5
Walk	1 minute		
Dead Hang p. 104	Hold as long as possible		

Fun Friday

Do something really playful today.

Super Saturday

Exercise	Distance/Time/Reps	Rest	Rounds
Piggy Back p. 126	20 meters		
Crouch to Sprint p. 118	20 seconds	2 minutes	
Repeat for 4 rounds total.			

Slow Down Sunday

Relax.

Level II: Week 4

Movement Monday	Paleo Circuit		
Exercise	**Distance/Time/Reps**	**Rest**	**Rounds**
Crouch to Sprint p. 118	20 meters		
Crab Walk left p. 96	5 meters		
Crab Walk right p. 96	5 meters		
Backward Bunny Hop p. 113	5 meters		
Feet-Together Toe Squat p. 121	10 reps	30 seconds	
Repeat for 30 minutes, rest as required.			

Tabata Tuesday	Tabata protocol (maximum intensity for 20 seconds, rest for 10 seconds)		
Exercise	**Distance/Time/Reps**	**Rest**	**Rounds**
Sprinting in Place p. 120	20 seconds	10 seconds	6
Walk	1 minute		
Burpee p. 89	20 seconds	10 seconds	6
Walk	1 minute		
Jump Rope p. 117	20 seconds	10 seconds	6
Walk	1 minute		
Get-Up/Stand-Up p. 83	20 seconds	10 seconds	6
Walk	1 minute		
Dead Hang p. 104	Hold as long as possible		

Walk Wednesday	Walk for 45 minutes. No power walking required. Be slow and mindful.

Tabata Thursday	Tabata protocol (maximum intensity for 20 seconds, rest for 10 seconds)		
Exercise	Distance/Time/Reps	Rest	Rounds
Jump Pull-Up p. 106	20 seconds	10 seconds	6
Walk	1 minute		
Parallel Bar Dip p. 82	20 seconds	10 seconds	6
Walk	1 minute		
Prisoner Squat p. 74	20 seconds	10 seconds	6
Walk	1 minute		
Push-Up p. 79	20 seconds	10 seconds	6
Walk	1 minute		
Hunter-Gatherer Squat p. 92	Hold as long as possible		

Fun Friday	Do something really playful today.

Super Saturday			
Exercise	Distance/Time/Reps	Rest	Rounds
Arm Plank p. 90	30 seconds		
Fireman's Carry p. 127	20 meters		
Crouch to Sprint p. 118	20 seconds	2 minutes	
Repeat for 3 rounds total.			

Slow Down Sunday	Relax.

LEVEL III

Level III: Week 1			
Movement Monday	Paleo Circuit		
Exercise	**Distance/Time/Reps**	**Rest**	**Rounds**
Crab Walk p. 96	30 meters		
Duck Walk p. 101	15 meters		
Cat Walk	25 meters		
Jump Pull-Up p. 106	15 reps		
Barefoot Walk Drill p. 70	30 seconds		
Repeat for 30 minutes; rest as required.			

Tabata Tuesday	Tabata protocol (maximum intensity for 20 seconds, rest for 10 seconds)		
Exercise	**Distance/Time/Reps**	**Rest**	**Rounds**
Burpee Push-Up p. 89	20 seconds	10 seconds	7
Walk	1 minute		
Crocodile Walk	20 seconds	10 seconds	7
Walk	1 minute		
Walking Lunge p. 76	20 seconds	10 seconds	7
Walk	1 minute		
Pull-Up p. 106	20 seconds	10 seconds	7
Rest 1 minute			
Hunter-Gatherer Squat p. 92	Hold as long as possible		

Walk Wednesday	Walk for 45 minutes. No power walking required. Be slow and mindful.

Tabata Thursday	Tabata protocol (maximum intensity for 20 seconds, rest for 10 seconds)		
Exercise	**Distance/Time/Reps**	**Rest**	**Rounds**
Jump Pull-Up p. 106	20 seconds	10 seconds	7
Walk	1 minute		
Crossover Knee p. 87	20 seconds	10 seconds	7
Walk	1 minute		
Sprinter's Lunge p. 76	20 seconds	10 seconds	7
Walk	1 minute		
Backward Cat Walk	20 seconds	10 seconds	7
Walk	1 minute		
Dead Hang p. 104	Hold as long as possible		
One-Legged Stand p. 123	Hold as long as possible		

Fun Friday	Do something really playful today.

Super Saturday			
Exercise	**Distance/Time/Reps**	**Rest**	**Rounds**
Dracula Carry p. 128	30 meters		
Barefoot Walk Drill p. 70	1 minute		
Crouch to Sprint p. 118	30 seconds		
Barefoot Walk Drill p. 70	2 minutes		
Repeat for 3 rounds total.			

Slow Down Sunday	Relax.

Level III: Week 2

Movement Monday	Paleo Circuit		
Exercise	**Distance/Time/Reps**	**Rest**	**Rounds**
Bunny Hops p. 113	10 meters		
Backward Bear Crawl p. 94	10 meters		
Power Pull-Up p. 106	2 reps		
Toddler Traverse p. 103	20 steps		
Backward Crab Walk p. 96	5 meters		
Walk	30 seconds		
Repeat for 30 minutes, active rest as required.			

Tabata Tuesday	Tabata protocol (maximum intensity for 20 seconds, rest for 10 seconds)		
Exercise	**Distance/Time/Reps**	**Rest**	**Rounds**
Tuck Jump p. 114	20 seconds	10 seconds	7
Walk	1 minute		
Salamander Press-Up p. 98	20 seconds	10 seconds	7
Walk	1 minute		
Crab Walk	20 seconds	10 seconds	7
Walk	1 minute		
Sprinter's Lunge p. 76	20 seconds	10 seconds	7
Rest 1 minute			
Crocodile Plank p. 91	Hold as long as possible		
Toe Stand p. 122	Hold as long as possible		

Walk Wednesday	Walk for 45 minutes. No power walking required. Be slow and mindful.

Tabata Thursday	Tabata protocol (maximum intensity for 20 seconds, rest for 10 seconds)		
Exercise	**Distance/Time/Reps**	**Rest**	**Rounds**
Power Pull-Up p. 106	20 seconds	10 seconds	7
Walk	1 minute		
Parallel Bar Dip p. 82	20 seconds	10 seconds	7
Walk	1 minute		
Squat Thrust p. 88	20 seconds	10 seconds	7
Walk	1 minute		
Double Unders p. 117	20 seconds	10 seconds	7
Walk	1 minute		
Rest 1 minute			
Gorilla Plank p. 90	Hold as long as possible		
Dead Hang p. 104	Hold as long as possible		

Fun Friday	Do something really playful today.

Super Saturday			
Exercise	**Distance/Time/Reps**	**Rest**	**Rounds**
Deadlift p. 129	10 reps		
Crouch to Sprint p. 118	30 seconds	2 minutes	
Repeat for 3 rounds total.			

Slow Down Sunday	Relax.

Level III: Week 3

Movement Monday	Paleo Circuit		
Exercise	**Distance/Time/Reps**	**Rest**	**Rounds**
Rabbit Walk p. 99	10 meters		
Muscle-Up p. 108	2 reps		
Bear Crawl p. 94	15 meters		
Toes-to-Bar p. 110	5 reps		
Kangaroo Jump p. 116	15 meters	30 seconds	
Repeat for 30 minutes, active rest as required.			

Tabata Tuesday	Tabata protocol (maximum intensity for 20 seconds, rest for 10 seconds)		
Exercise	**Distance/Time/Reps**	**Rest**	**Rounds**
Chin-Over p. 105	20 seconds	10 seconds	8
Walk	1 minute		
Crouch to Sprint p. 118	20 seconds	10 seconds	8
Walk	1 minute		
Clock Push-Up p. 80	20 seconds	10 seconds	8
Walk	1 minute		
Sprinter's Lunge p. 76	20 seconds	10 seconds	8
Walk	1 minute		
Dead Hang p. 104	Hold as long as possible		
Heel Stand p. 122	Hold as long as possible		

Walk Wednesday	Walk for 45 minutes. No power walking required. Be slow and mindful.

Tabata Thursday	Tabata protocol (maximum intensity for 20 seconds, rest for 10 seconds)		
Exercise	**Distance/Time/Reps**	**Rest**	**Rounds**
Push-Up p. 79	20 seconds	10 seconds	8
Walk	1 minute		
Prisoner Squat p. 74	20 seconds	10 seconds	8
Walk	1 minute		
Double Unders p. 117	20 seconds	10 seconds	8
Walk	1 minute		
Bear Crawl p. 94	20 seconds	10 seconds	8
Rest 1 minute			
Crocodile Plank p. 91	Hold as long as possible		
Reverse Plank p. 91	Hold as long as possible		

Fun Friday	Do something really playful today.

Super Saturday			
Exercise	**Distance/Time/Reps**	**Rest**	**Rounds**
Car Push p. 135	75 meters		
Push Press p. 131	10		
Crouch to Sprint p. 118	20 seconds	2 minute	
Repeat for 4 rounds total.			

Slow Down Sunday	Relax.

Level III: Week 4

Movement Monday	Paleo Circuit		
Exercise	**Distance/Time/Reps**	**Rest**	**Rounds**
Crouch to Sprint p. 118	10 meters		
Crab Walk left p. 96	5 meters		
Muscle-Up p. 108	2 reps		
Crab Walk right p. 96	5 meters		
Backward Bunny Hop p. 113	5 meters	30 seconds	
Repeat for 30 minutes, rest as required.			

Tabata Tuesday	Tabata protocol (maximum intensity for 20 seconds, rest for 10 seconds)		
Exercise	**Distance/Time/Reps**	**Rest**	**Rounds**
Squat Jump p. 115	20 seconds	10 seconds	8
Walk	1 minute		
Rabbit Walk p. 99	20 seconds	10 seconds	8
Walk	1 minute		
Jump Rope p. 117	20 seconds	10 seconds	8
Walk	1 minute		
Get-Up/Stand-Up p. 83	20 seconds	10 seconds	8
Walk	1 minute		
Dead Hang p. 104	Hold as long as possible		
Arm Plank p. 90	Hold as long as possible		

Walk Wednesday	Walk for 45 minutes. No power walking required. Be slow and mindful.

Tabata Thursday	Tabata protocol (maximum intensity for 20 seconds, rest for 10 seconds)		
Exercise	**Distance/Time/Reps**	**Rest**	**Rounds**
Jump Pull-Up p. 106	20 seconds	10 seconds	8
Walk	1 minute		
Chair Dip p. 81	20 seconds	10 seconds	8
Walk	1 minute		
Prisoner Squat p. 74	20 seconds	10 seconds	8
Walk	1 minute		
Push-Up p. 79	20 seconds	10 seconds	8
Rest 1 minute			
Wall Sit p. 92	Hold as long as possible		
Gorilla Plank p. 90	Hold as long as possible		

Fun Friday	Do something really playful today.

Super Saturday			
Exercise	**Distance/Time/Reps**	**Rest**	**Rounds**
Fireman's Carry Squat p. 74	3–5 reps	1 minute	
Crouch to Sprint p. 118	20 seconds	2 minutes	
Repeat for 5 rounds total.			

Slow Down Sunday	Relax.

THE EXERCISES

Preparation (more than just a warm-up!)

In addition to preparing our bodies for movement, we'll use this section to keep our workouts playful. The emphasis is on smooth, controlled movement, staying within a controlled range of motion that gradually increases as your muscles and joints loosen and warm up. Think of it as oiling the joints and regaining your natural right to freedom of movement.

Before each workout, perform each of the following activities for 1–2 minutes each for a total of 5–10 minutes of warm-up. Unlike conventional mobility drills, our focus as always will be on full-body movements.

SLOW-MO

Pick a movement such as a crawl, walk or virtual throw and perform as slowly and as exaggerated as possible.

BAREFOOT WALK DRILL

This naturally stretches and strengthens your lower legs to prevent injury. Use this opportunity to get used to moving without shoes again and to strengthen the muscles of the foot and ankle.

- Walk at differing tempos on your heels, balls of your feet and tiptoes.
- Walk on the insides and outsides of your feet.
- Walk with differing amounts of pressure, from very hard to very light.
- Alternate between bearing more weight on the forward foot, and then more on the back.

HOT COALS

Walk on the balls of your feet as if you were walking on hot coals. Challenge your balance and stability with each step. Be as quiet as you can and softly plant your feet.

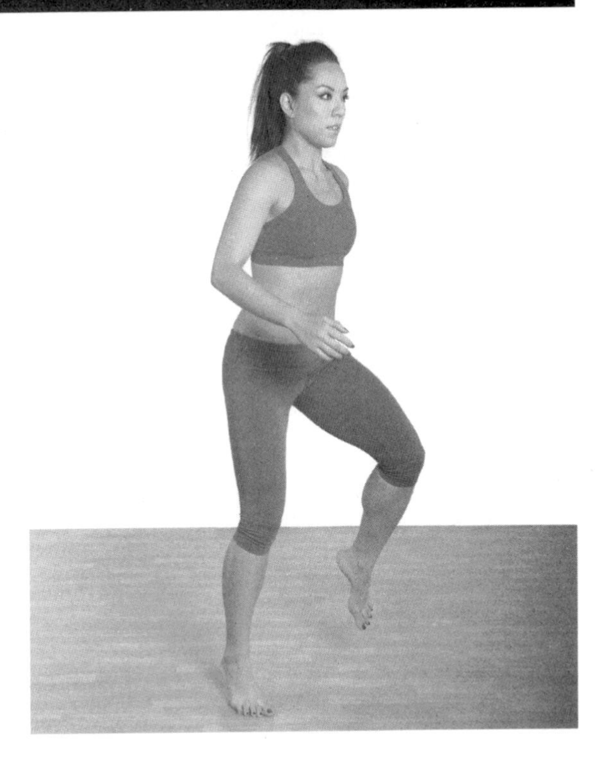

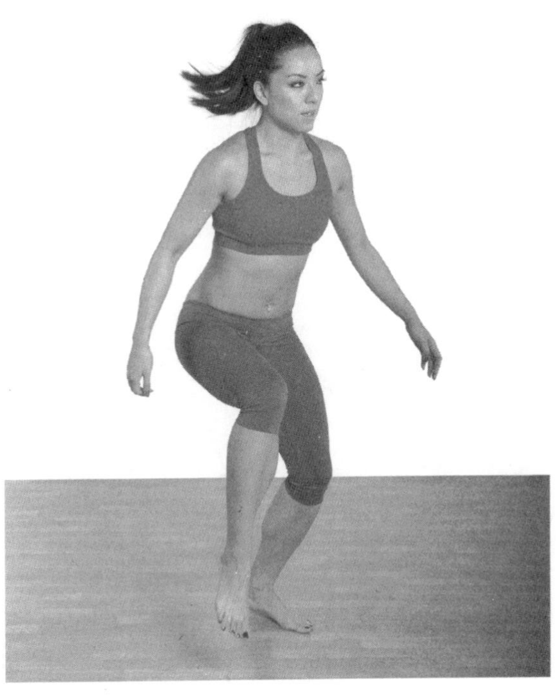

VIRTUAL JUMP ROPE

Perform a skipping (jump rope) motion without a rope. Do as many combinations as possible: single leg, high knee, alternative leg, crossovers, etc. Go wild and use your imagination.

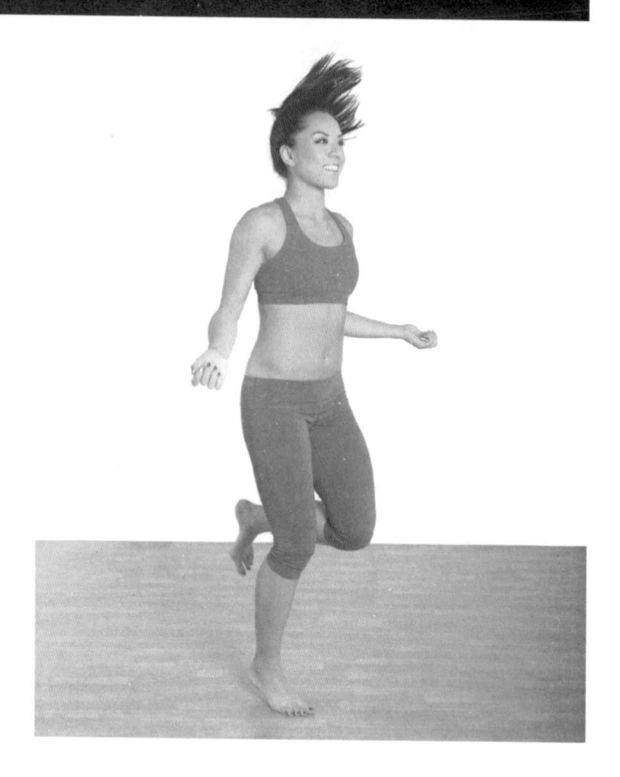

VIRTUAL THROW

Perform a throw without an object and do as many throw variations as possible: single hand, both hands, overhead, javelin, etc. Again, imagination is key to take your body through as many combinations and positions as possible.

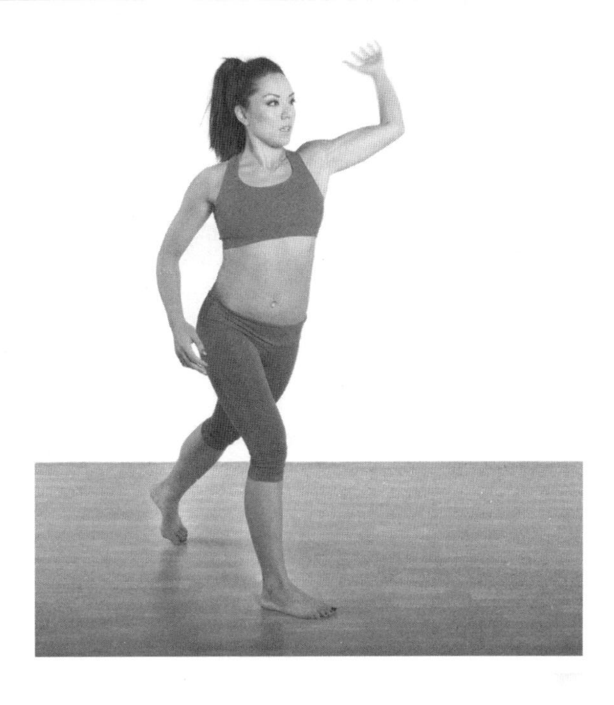

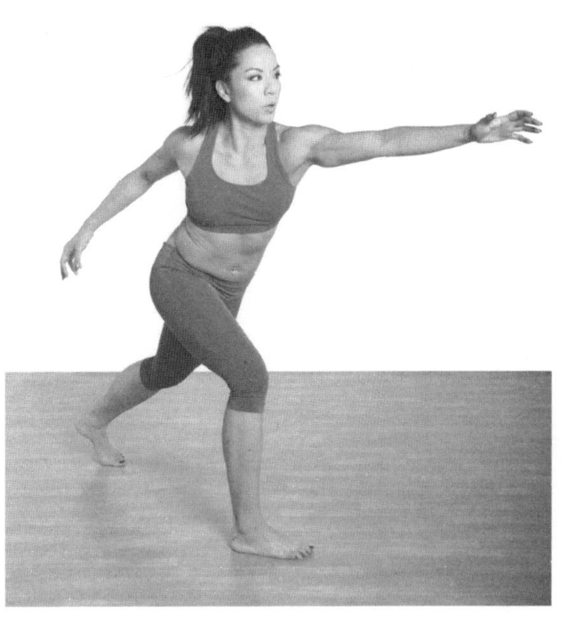

Fundamental Movements

These moves are the foundation of the Paleo Fitness *program. Here you'll build a base on which to increase your overall fitness in terms of aerobic capacity, strength, flexibility, and mental and physical endurance. Don't mistake these moves as beginner exercises or as being simple to do. When you use correct form they'll challenge you regardless of fitness level or how long you've trained.*

SQUAT

The squat is a functional movement pattern based on sitting down and standing up. It's an essential movement that will protect against injury as well as rehabilitate and maintain the integrity of your back, hips, knees and ankles. For some reason the word "squat" strikes fear in individuals who may be concerned about the impact on their knees. Just think of it as sitting down and standing up; if those cause discomfort, then all the more reason to work on this most fundamental of movements. We're not aiming for the "Jane Fonda aerobics" squat with little range of motion, but squats of significantly higher quality, difficulty and depth. This may take some time to achieve due to a lack of flexibility or strength but it's the perfect antidote to all the sitting in a chair we do.

1 Stand with your feet shoulder-width apart and feet slightly turned out.

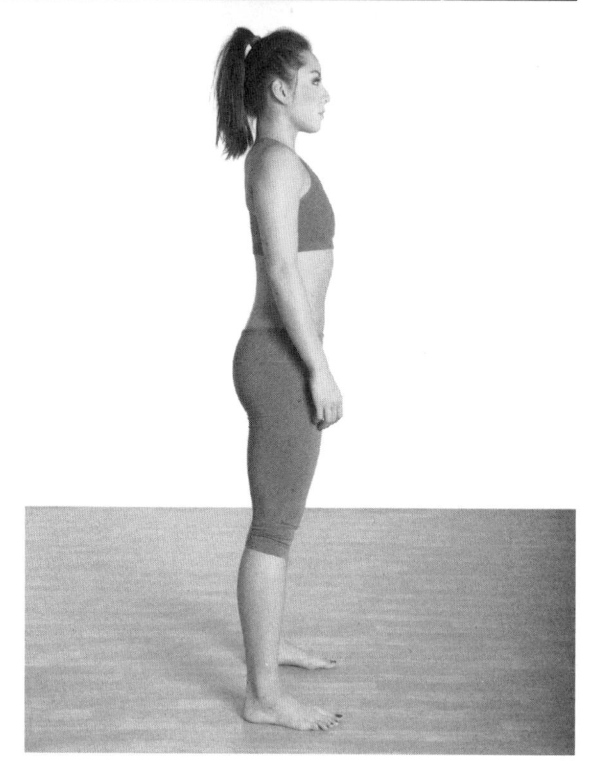

1

2 Exhale, bend your knees and move your butt down as though you were going to sit back into a chair; lift your arms up and out to assist with balance. Keep your head up in a neutral position and accentuate the arch of your lower back (lumbar curve) by keeping your chest high and shoulders back. Keep your midsection tight. As you descend, let your knees track over your feet without letting them roll inside or outside the feet. Keep as much pressure on the heels as possible and stay off the balls of the feet. Keep your torso elongated, avoiding any exaggerated forward lean. Viewed from the side, your ears should travel down in a straight line rather than move forward.

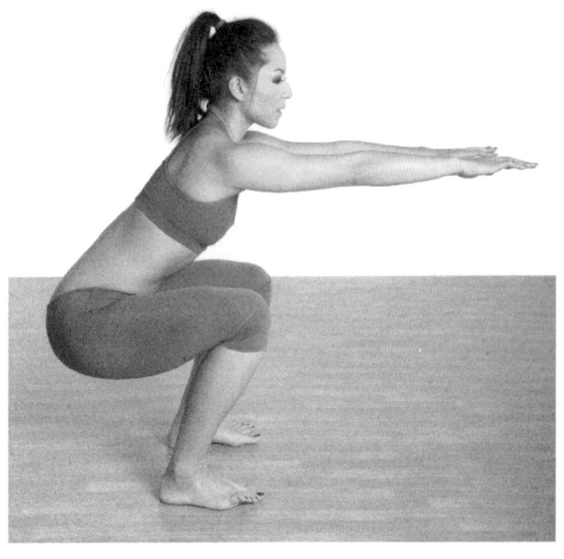

2

Stop when the crease of the hip is below the knee, just below parallel to the floor. Don't lose the lumbar curve when in the bottom position; continue to keep your heels flat on the ground.

Inhale and reverse the movement on exactly the same path as you descended to stand up, without any forward lean. The whole body should be involved with this movement in a controlled fashion, regardless of speed. At the top of the movement stand as tall as possible.

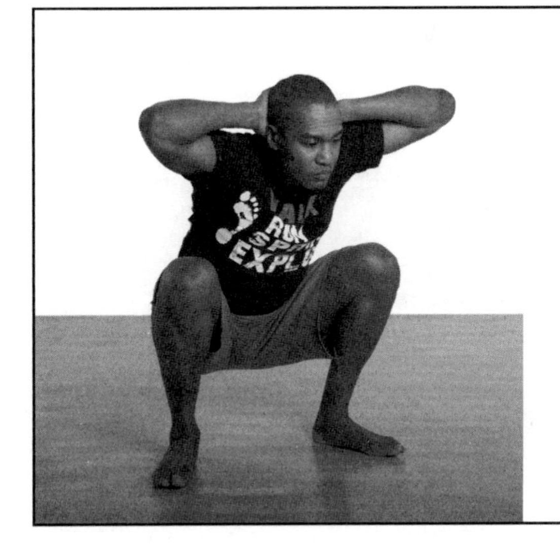

PRISONER SQUAT VARIATION: This is identical to the standard squat except you clasp your hands together behind your head throughout the movement. Be careful not to pull your head forward as this causes unneeded stress on the neck muscles. Keep your elbows back and away from your body and squeeze your shoulder blades throughout the movement to work the upper back; pretend as if you're gripping a pencil between your shoulder blades. It's easier for the torso to lean forward during this move than in the standard squat, so work even harder to keep your torso as upright as possible.

LUNGE

The lunge is an advanced walking exercise, albeit with a longer stride. This trains you unilaterally (one side independently from the other), which improves balance and coordination. It also forces you to open your hip flexors, which are tight for many who spend significant time sitting.

1 Stand tall with your feet shoulder-width apart and your arms hanging at your sides.

2 Take a large step forward with your left foot, bend both knees and drop your hips straight down until both knees are bent 90 degrees. Your right knee should almost be touching the ground with your right toes on the ground behind you. Keep your midsection tight and your back, neck and hips straight at all times during this movement.

Pushing up with your left leg, straighten both knees and return to starting position.

Repeat with the other leg.

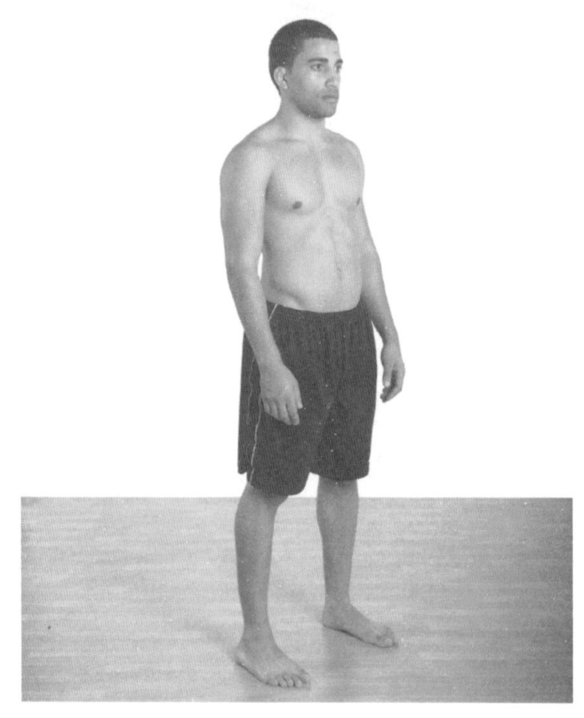

1

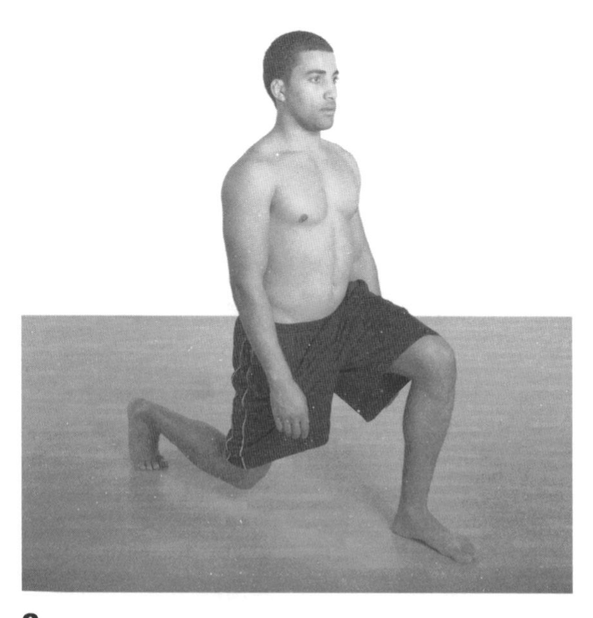

2

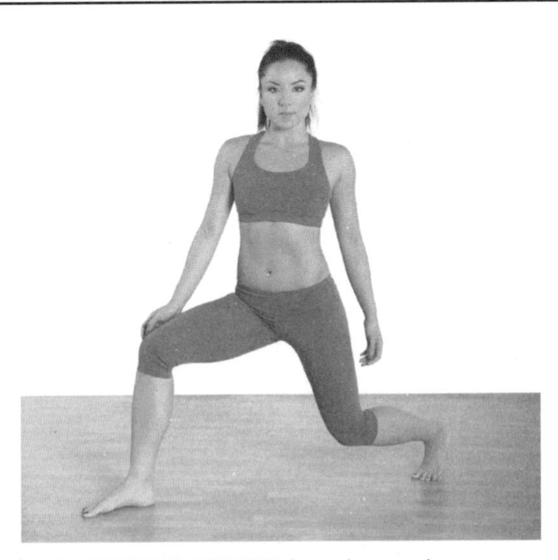

CLOCKWORK LUNGE: Imagine you're standing in the middle of a clock face on the ground with your nose pointing at 12 o'clock. Step forward into a lunge with your right leg. Pause, then step back to center. Turn so your nose is pointing at 1 o'clock and repeat. Continue around the clock face until you reach 6 o'clock. Repeat with the left leg lunging forward, but this time work counterclockwise starting at 11 o'clock, working backward to 10 o'clock and so on back to 6 o'clock. Make sure your torso and hips are always facing 12 o'clock as much as possible.

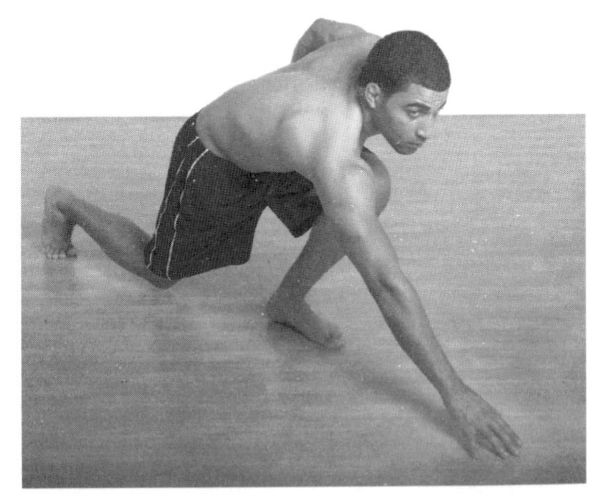

LUNGE WITH REACH: As you step forward and drop your hips into the lunge, lean forward on your left leg as far as you can. You may need to support yourself on the ball of your right foot. With your torso leaning on your left thigh, reach as far as you can and, if possible, touch the ground, aiming for a virtual (or real) target on the ground.

REVERSE LUNGE: Rather than stepping forward, take big backward steps on each side.

WALKING LUNGE: Push up from the bottom of the squat with your left leg. Take a large step forward past your right foot so that your right toes are balanced on the ground behind you. Drop your hips down until both knees are bent 90 degrees.

THRUSTER

1 Stand with your feet shoulder-width apart and feet slightly turned out. Perform a Squat (page 74).

2 From the bottom position of the squat, as you press up through your heels into the top position, raise your arms forward in an arc until your hands are above your head and reach your fingertips toward the ceiling to activate your shoulders and upper back.

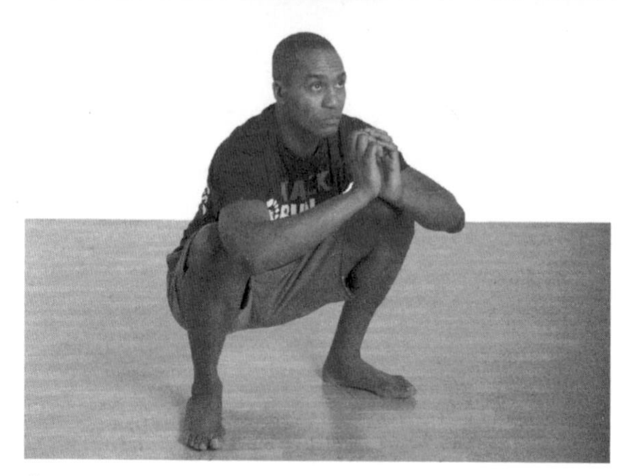

1

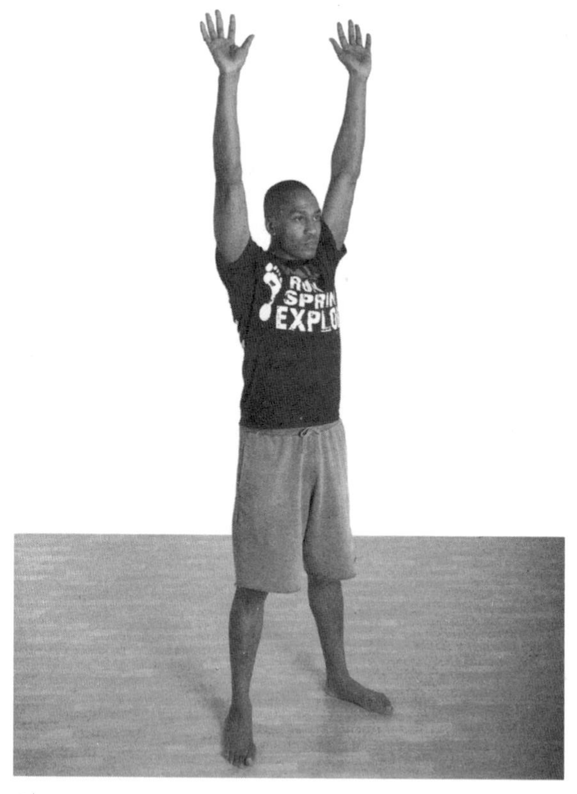

2

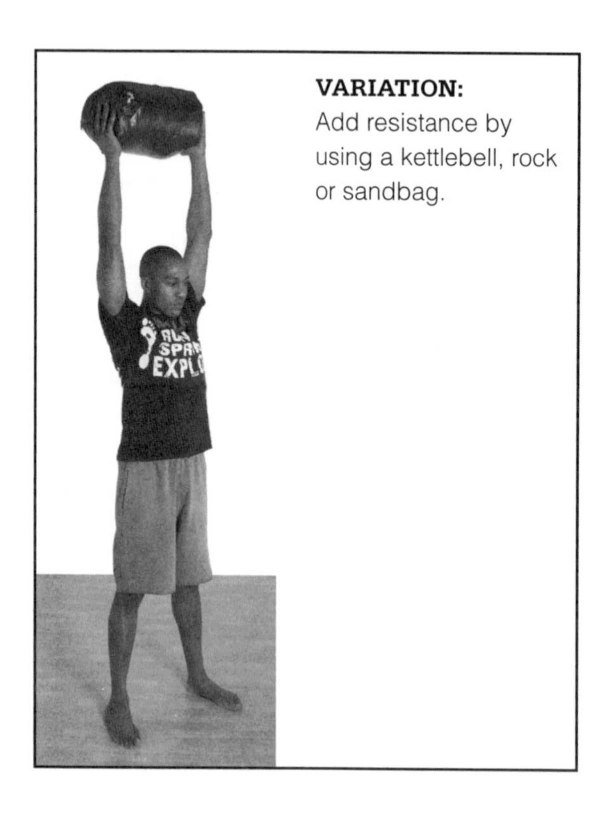

VARIATION:
Add resistance by using a kettlebell, rock or sandbag.

STANDING PUSH-UP

This movement is an alternative to traditional push-ups on the floor. Focus on your arms doing the work rather than just moving your torso.

1 Start in a standing position with your feet shoulder-width apart. Hunch over to place your hands on your slightly bent knees, with your elbows slightly bent.

2 Inhale and lower your upper body as far as you can by bending your arms only, not using your torso or back.

Exhale and push back up to starting position using only your arms and chest.

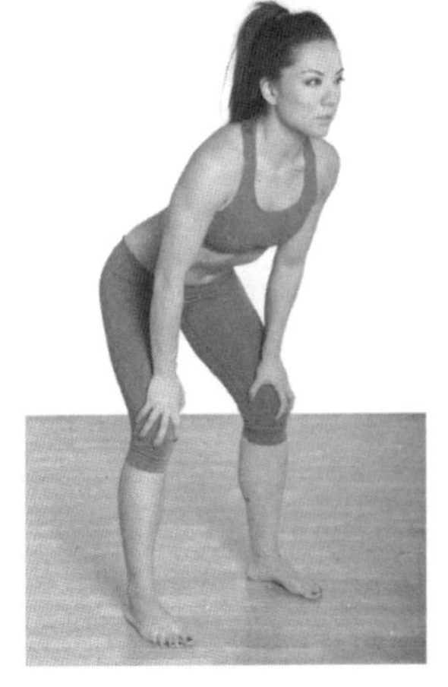

1

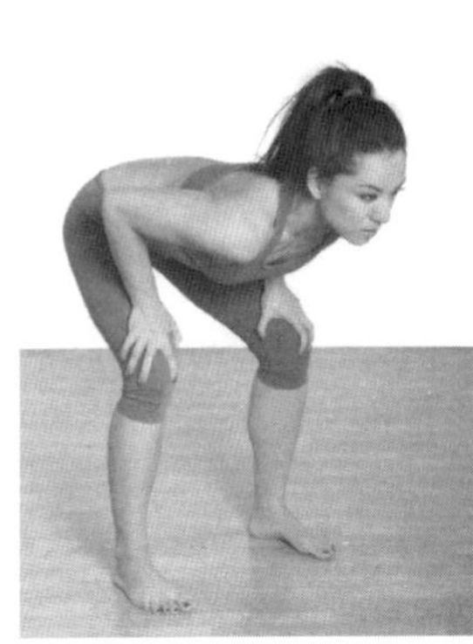

2

PUSH-UP

1 Place your hands on the ground approximately shoulder-width apart, with your fingers pointing straight ahead and your arms straight. Step your feet back until your body forms a straight line from head to toe. Keep your feet together and hold your midsection and back tight.

2 Inhale as you lower your torso to the ground and focus on keeping your elbows as close to your sides as possible. Stop when your chest and body touch the floor.

Using your whole body, exhale and push your torso back up to starting position.

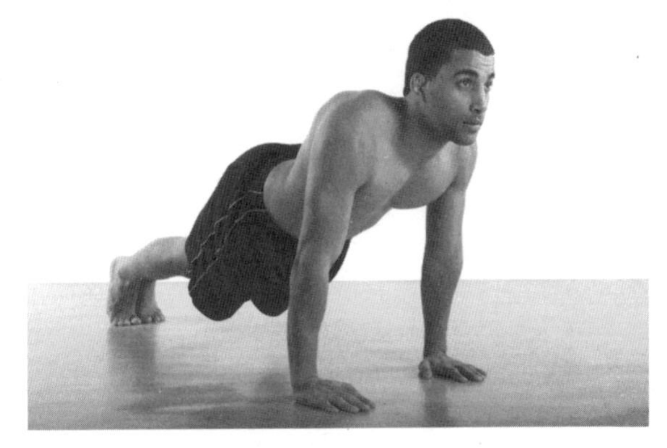

1

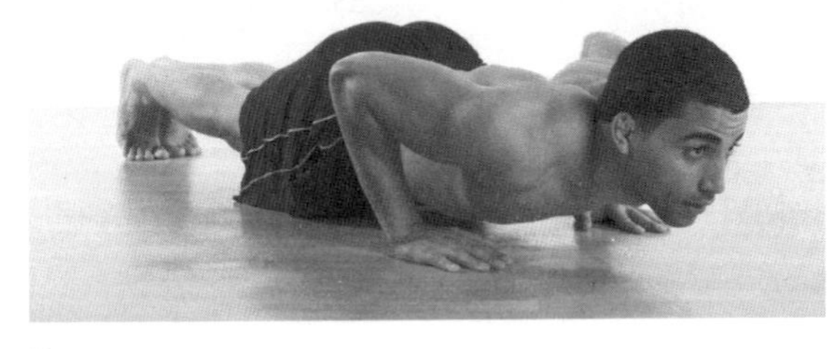

2

> **VARIATION:**
> Push-ups can also be done with the hands set wide apart or narrow and close together.

CLOCK PUSH-UP

1–2 Start in a push-up position (see page 79), with your left arm directly below your shoulder and your right arm slightly in front. Imagine the right arm is at 12 o'clock. Complete a push-up in this position.

3–4 Move you're the right arm to 1 o'clock and perform another push-up.

Then move to 3 o'clock and do a push-up, and finally 5 o'clock and do a push-up. Repeat on the other side with the left arm starting at 12 o'clock and working counterclockwise to 11 o'clock, then 9 o'clock, then 7 o'clock.

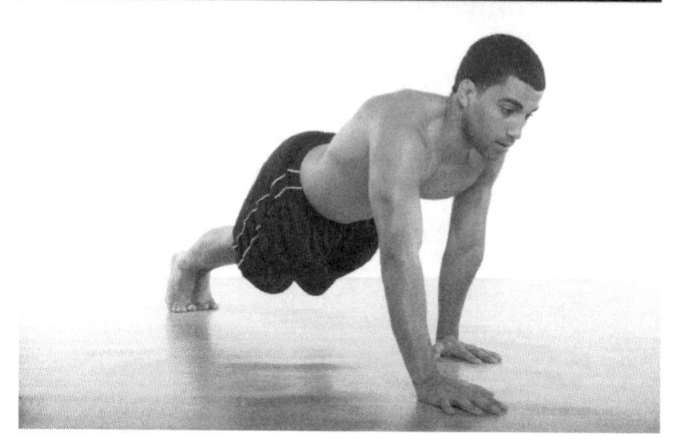

1

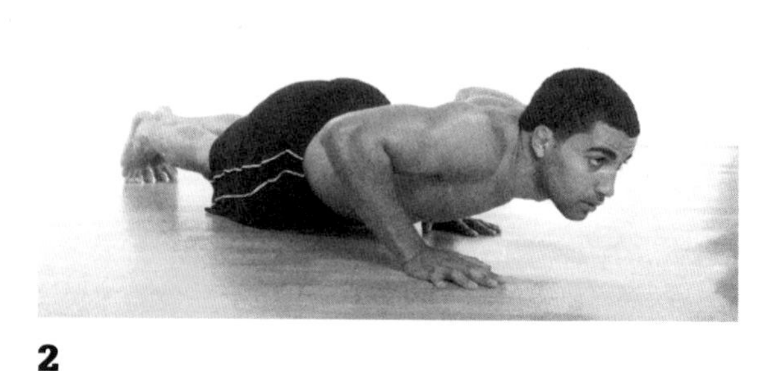

2

3

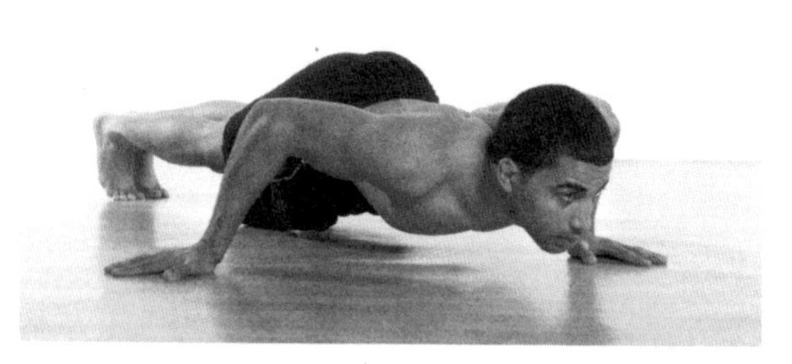

4

CHAIR DIP

1 Sit on a chair, sofa, bench or similar with your hands next to your hips. Lift up onto your hands and push your hips forward off the chair. Your feet should be up on your heels.

2 Bend your elbows 90 degrees and lower your hips toward the floor, keeping close to the chair and your back as straight as possible. Don't shrug your shoulders; keep them down during the whole movement.

Push back up.

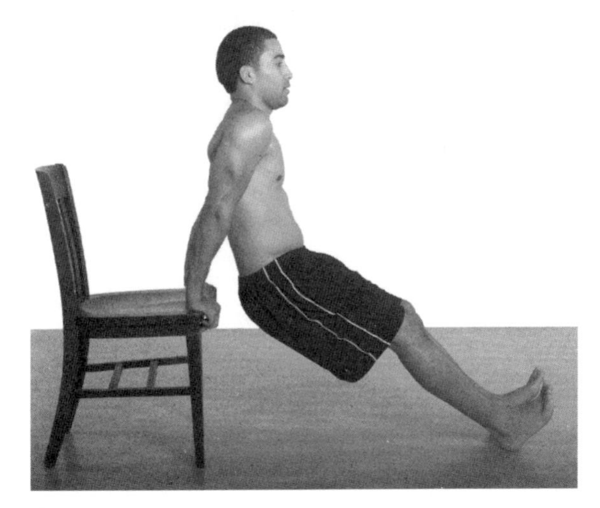

1

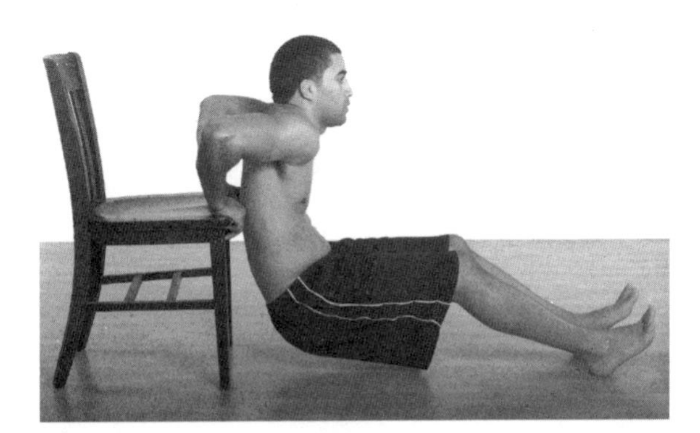

2

VARIATIONS: To make the move easier, bend your knees and bring your feet closer to the chair with your feet flat. To make it more difficult, straighten your legs. For an advanced version, place your feet on another chair or raise one leg during the movement.

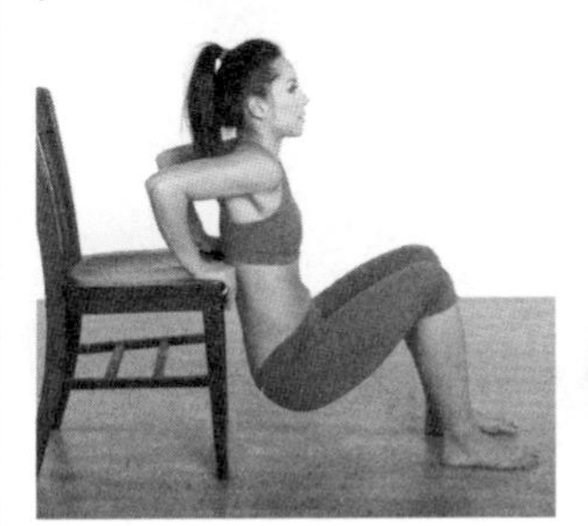

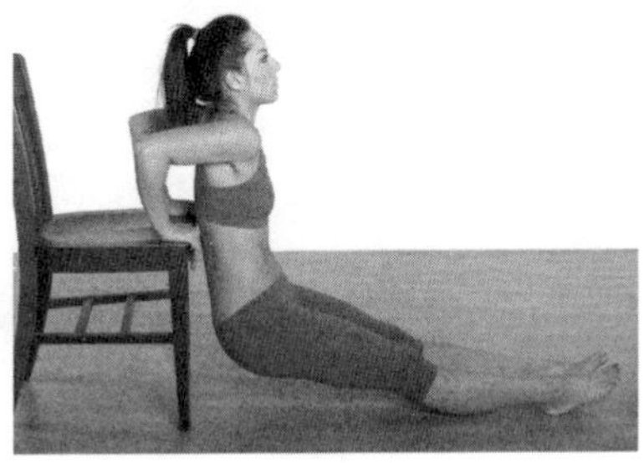

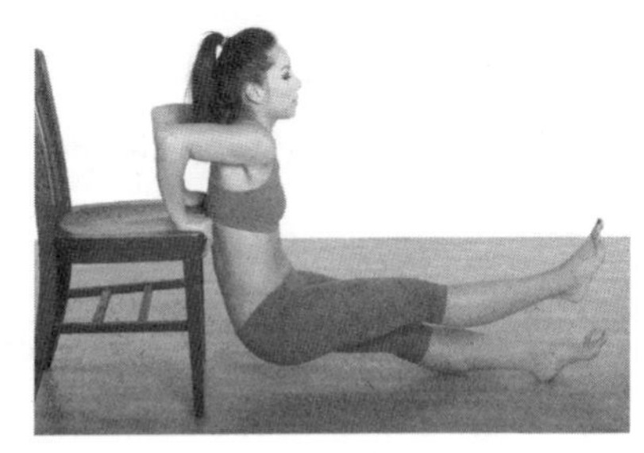

PARALLEL BAR DIP

1 Position yourself between two parallel bars. Hold onto the bars with your arms extended and feet slightly off the ground.

2 Lower your chest by bending your elbows until they reach a 90-degree angle.

Straighten your arms to return to starting position.

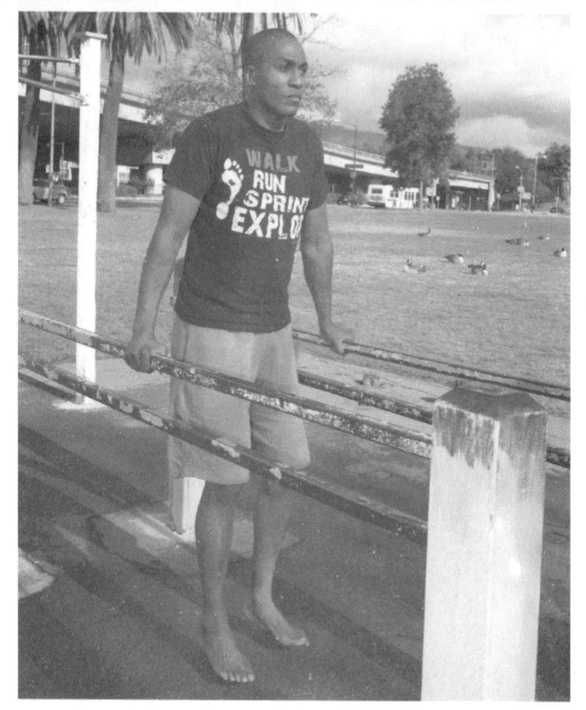

1

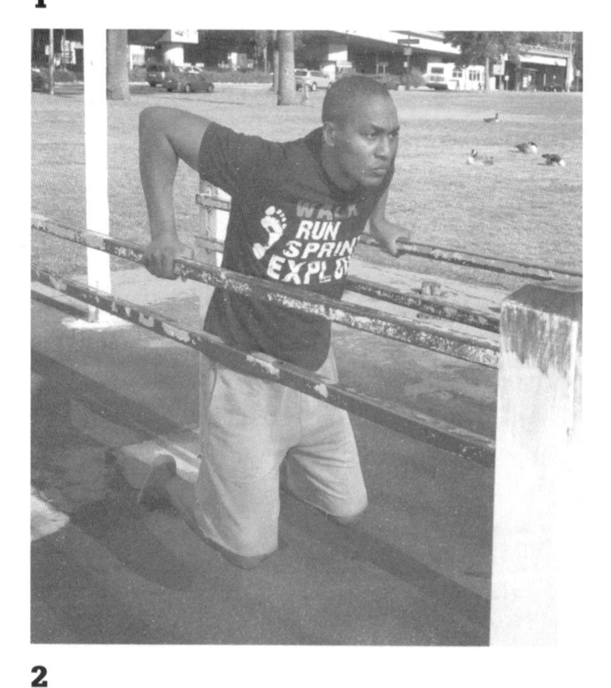

2

GET-UP/STAND-UP

1 Stand tall with your feet shoulder-width apart and your arms hanging at your sides.

2 Sit down on the ground. For additional support you can use one or both hands.

3 As soon as you sit down fully, stand straight back up (imagine sitting on a hot plate!). Push off with one or both hands. Do this as quickly as possible!

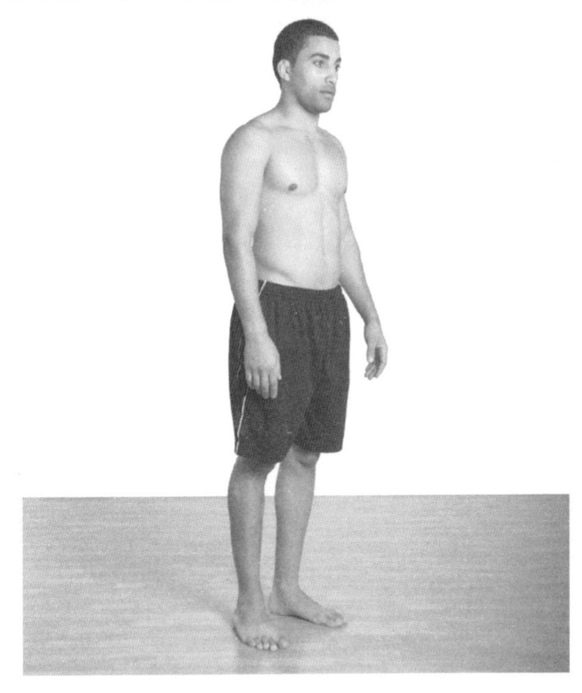

1

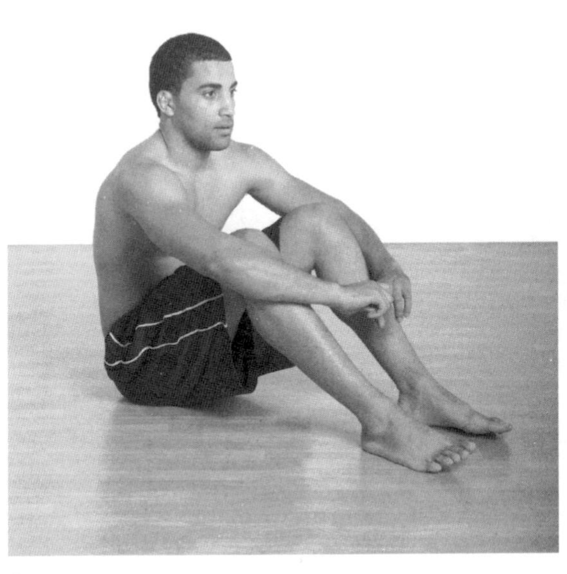

2

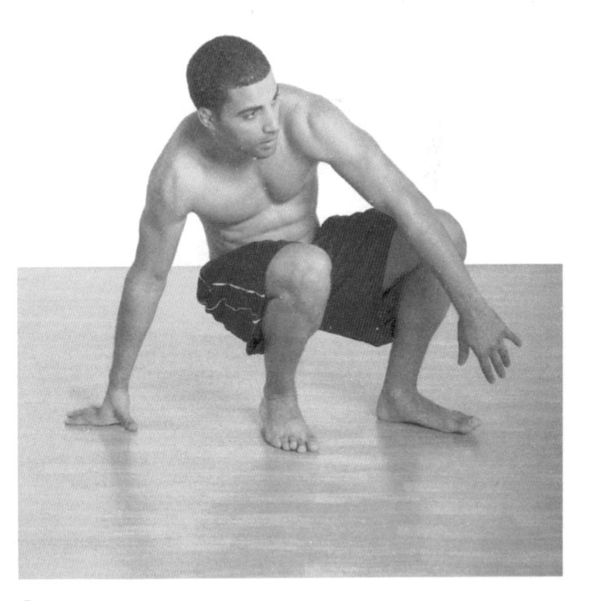

3

RESISTED ARM PRESS

1 Stand tall with your feet shoulder-width apart. Make a fist with your left hand and bend your left arm. Rest your right hand on top of your left fist.

2–4 Keeping your right hand on the left, press your left hand up, overhead and down to the opposite shoulder. Apply enough resistance for the movement to be just about possible. Keep a natural breathing pattern.

Take your arm back overhead to starting position. Switch hand positions.

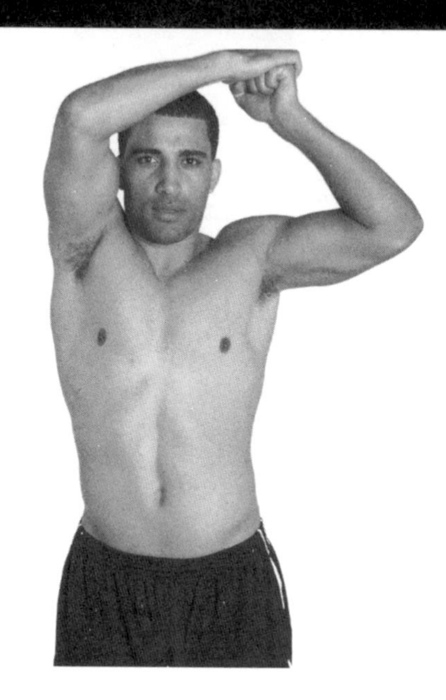

1

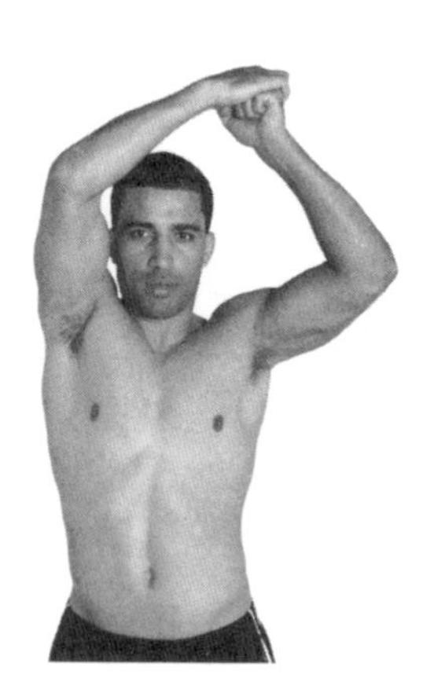

2

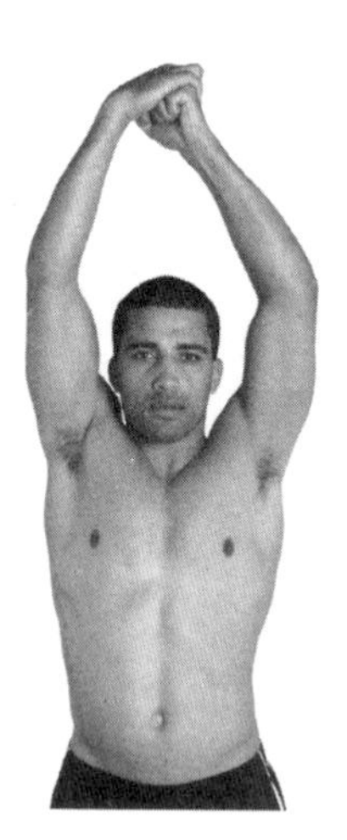

3

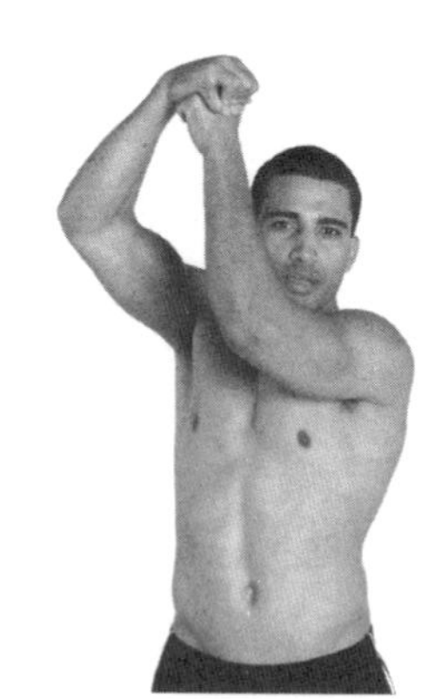

4

BACK EXTENSION

1 Lie face down and place your hands alongside your body. Contract your midsection and keep it tight throughout.

2 Squeeze from your lower back to lift your chest a few inches off the ground. Pause briefly.

Lower to starting position.

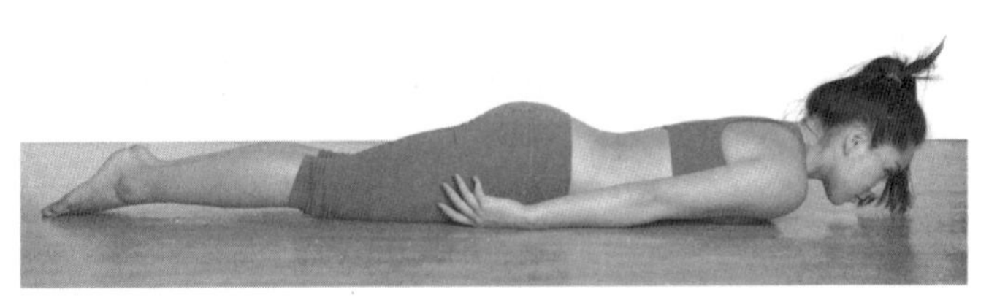

1

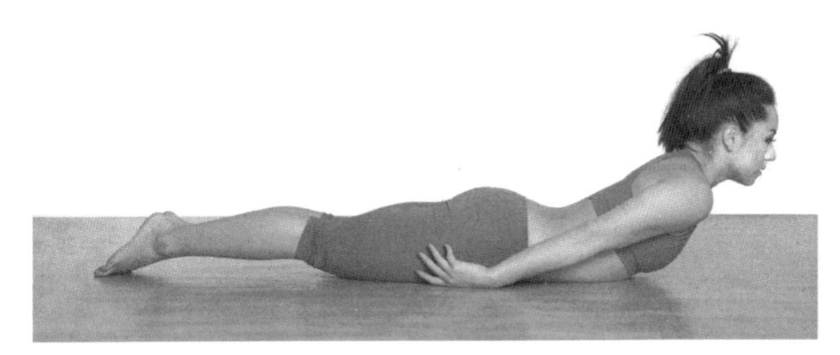

2

VARIATIONS: To make it more difficult, place your hands behind your head and squeeze your shoulder blades together as you lift your chest up off the ground. For an even more advanced move, lift your legs off the ground as you lift your chest, keeping your feet together.

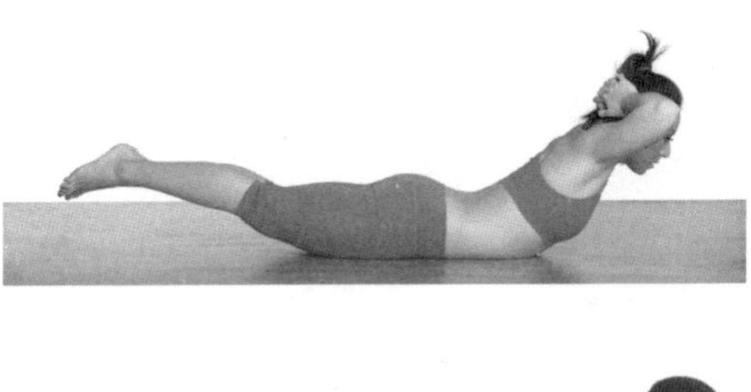

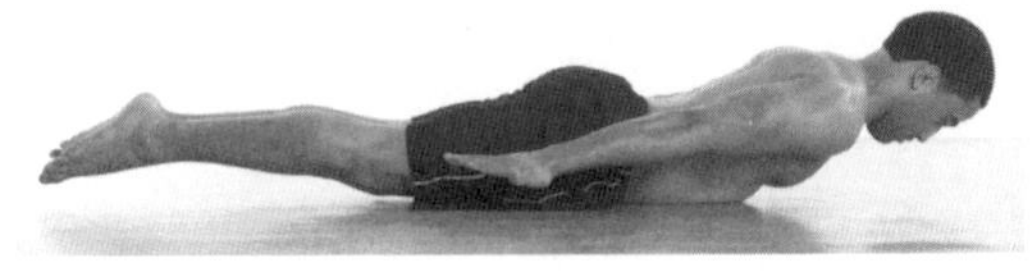

Speed/Coordination Development

SHIN GRAB SIT-UP

1 Lie on your back with your arms behind your head and legs fully extended.

2 Without letting your feet touch the floor, curl up and bring your knees into your chest, simultaneously wrapping your arms around your shins.

Return to starting position.

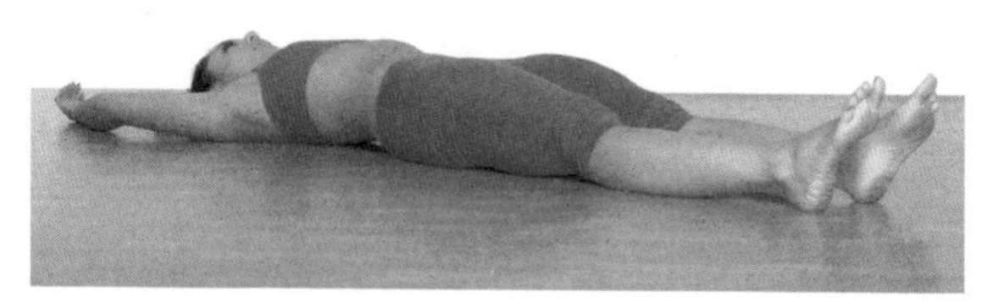

1

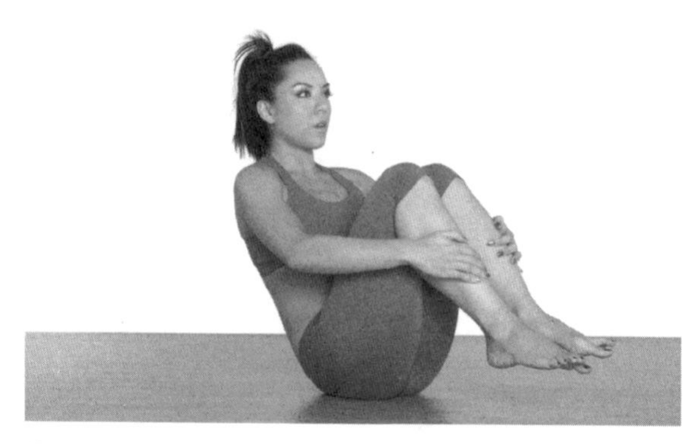

2

CROSSOVER KNEE

1 Stand tall with your feet together. Clasp your hands together behind your head throughout.

2 Raise your right knee and twist your torso to touch it with your left elbow.

3 Return to starting position, raise your left knee, and touch with your right elbow.

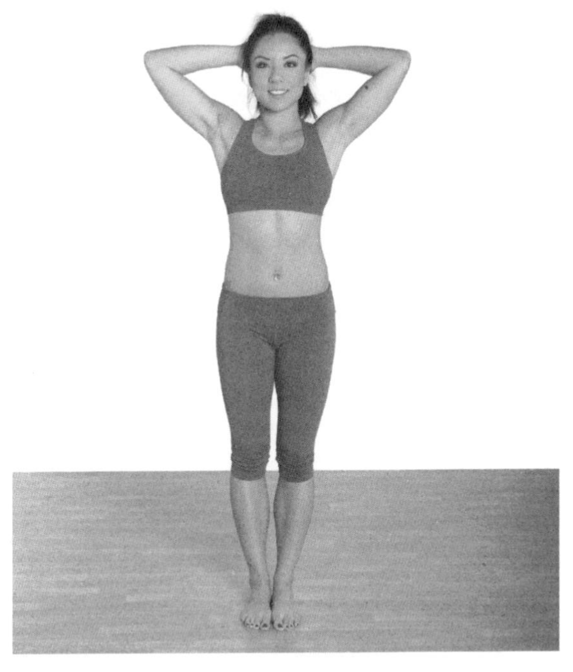

1

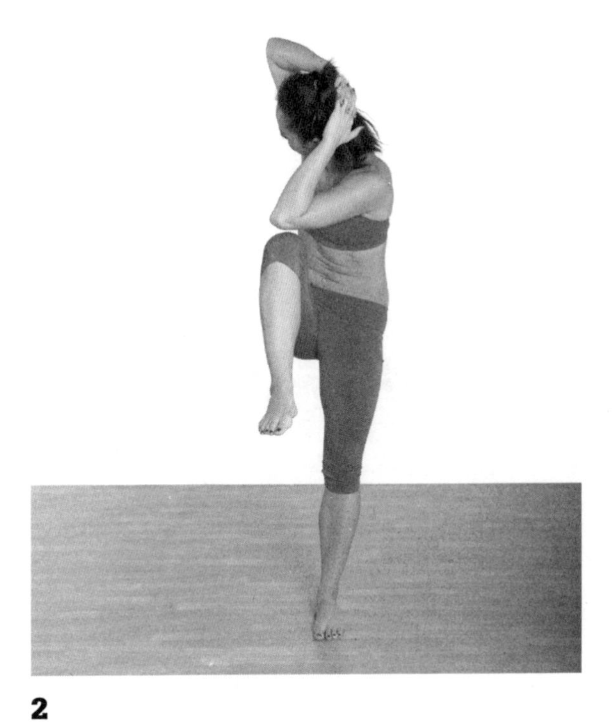

2

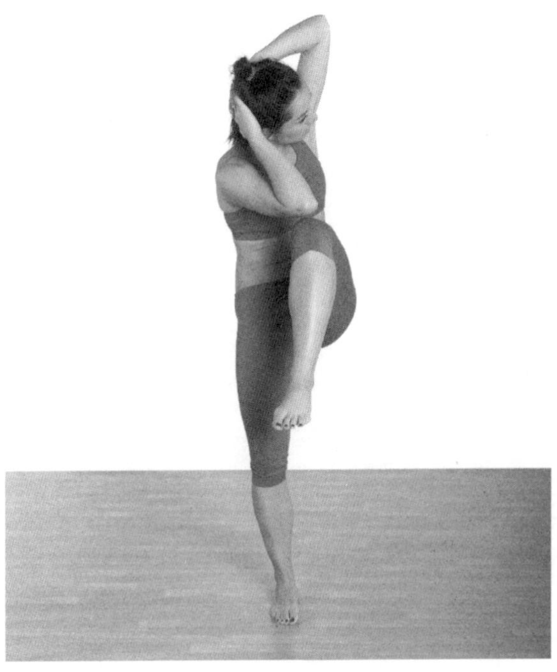

3

SQUAT THRUST

1 Start in a crouched position with your hands on the ground on either side of your body.

2 Keep your hands where they are and kick your legs back into arm plank position (page 90) in one quick motion.

3 Jump your feet back to starting position.

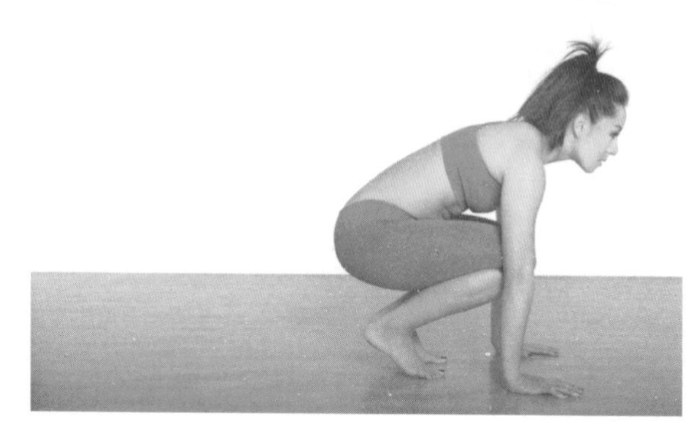

1

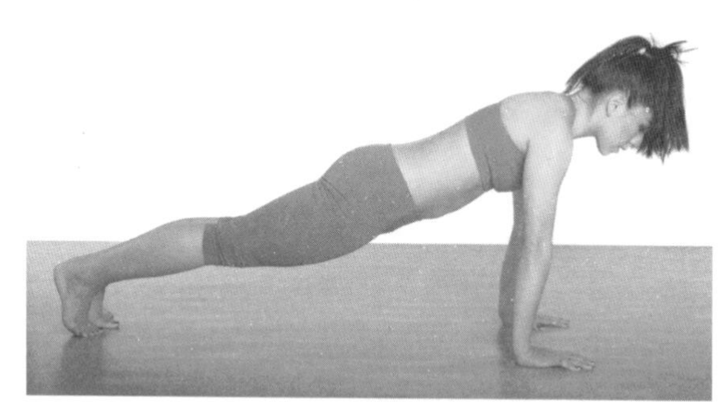

2

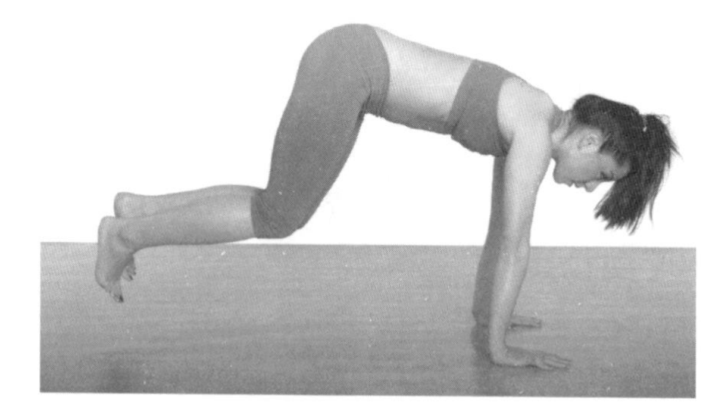

3

BURPEE

1 Stand tall with your feet shoulder-width apart and your arms hanging at your sides.

2 Drop into a crouched position with your hands on the ground on either side of your body.

3 Keep your hands where they are and kick your feet back into arm plank position (page 90) in one quick motion.

4 Jump your feet back to the crouched position in one quick motion.

5 Jump straight up, landing softly.

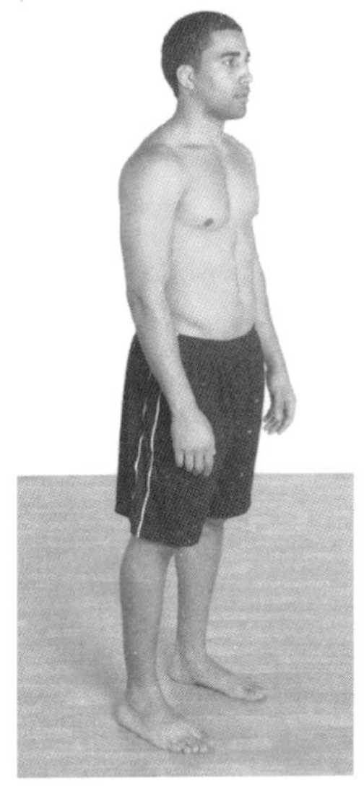

1

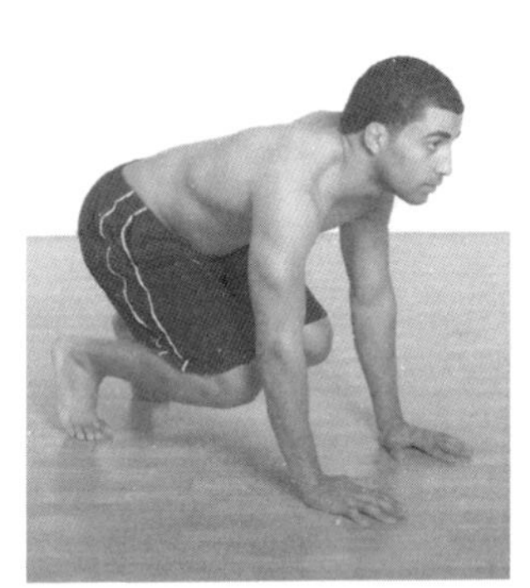

2

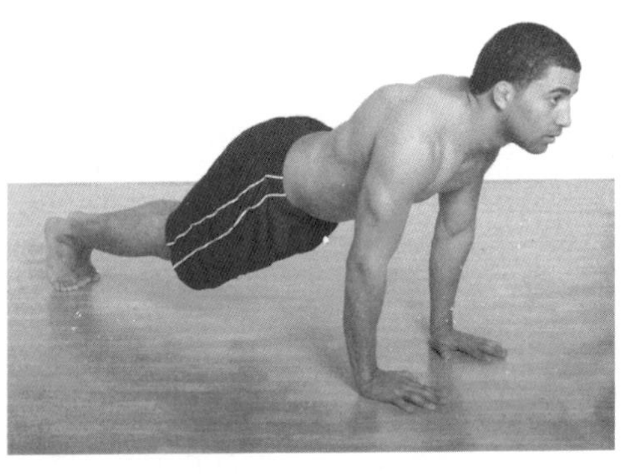

3

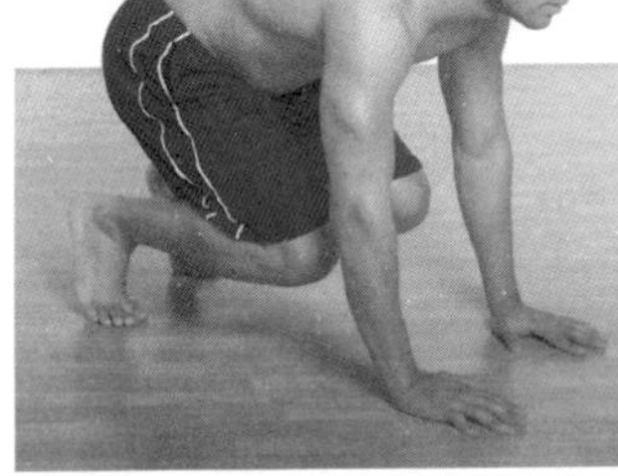

4

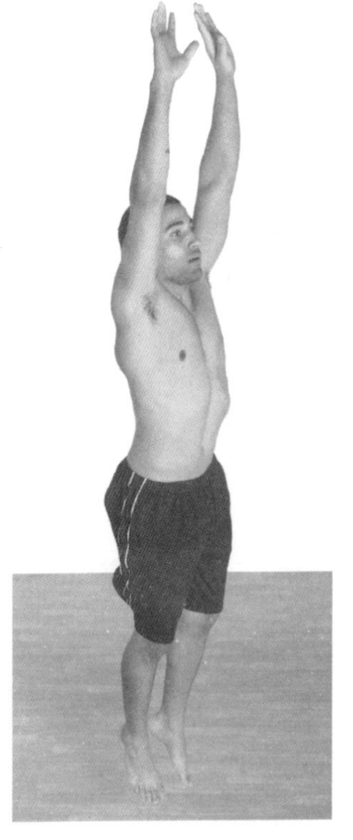

5

BURPEE PUSH-UP VARIATION: Perform a regular burpee but add a push-up once in the arm plank position.

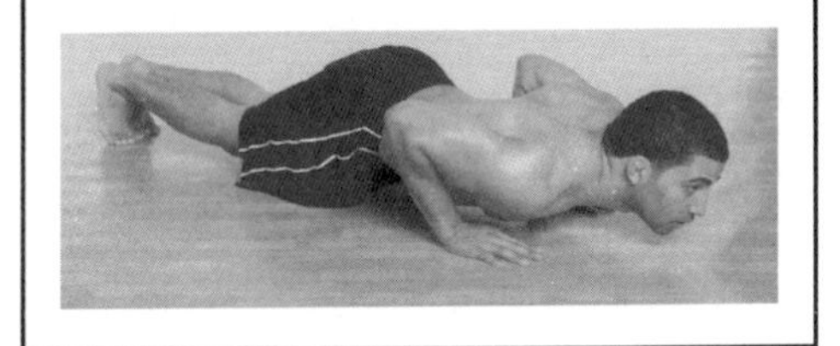

Stationary Moves (Isometric)

These stationary "moves" are isometric, meaning they're static exercises where the muscles are contracting but there's no movement at the joint. They're useful for building strength around the joint and improving posture and focus.

ARM PLANK

Place your hands on the ground approximately shoulder-width apart, making sure your fingers point straight ahead and your arms are straight but your elbows not locked. Step your feet back until your body forms a straight line from head to toe. Keep your feet together. Tighten your midsection to keep your spine from sagging; don't sink into your shoulders. Keep a natural breathing pattern.

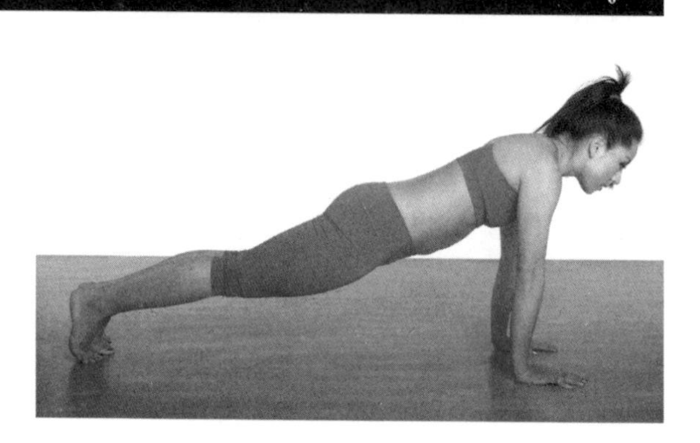

GORILLA PLANK

Start in a crouched position and drop onto all fours with your hands directly under your shoulders. Fully extend your arms, then rise up onto the balls of your feet. Your knees should be directly under your hips and arms in line with your shoulders. Make sure your hips and knees are not too high off the ground. Maintain an arched back throughout.

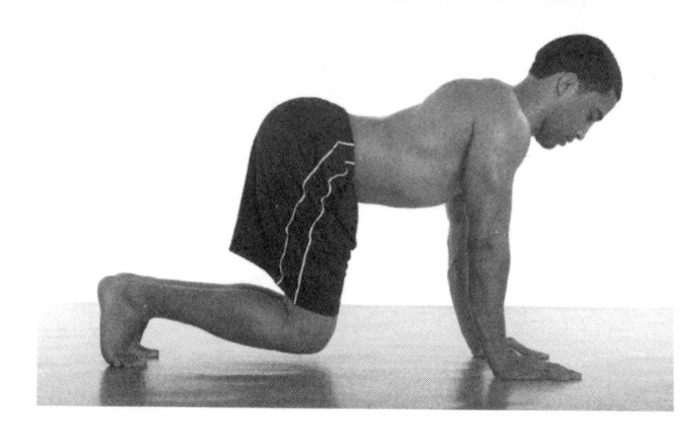

REVERSE PLANK

In this plank you're facing upward.

1 Start from a seated position with your legs extended in front of you and your hands slightly behind and outside your hips.

2 Slowly straighten your arms and lift your hips until your body forms a straight line from heels to shoulders, with your head in line with your body.

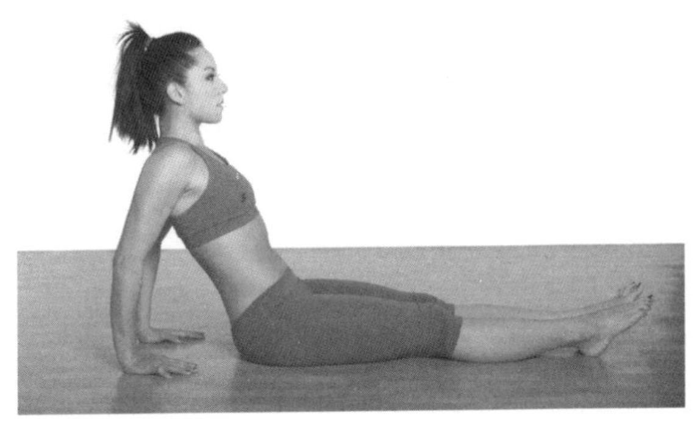

1

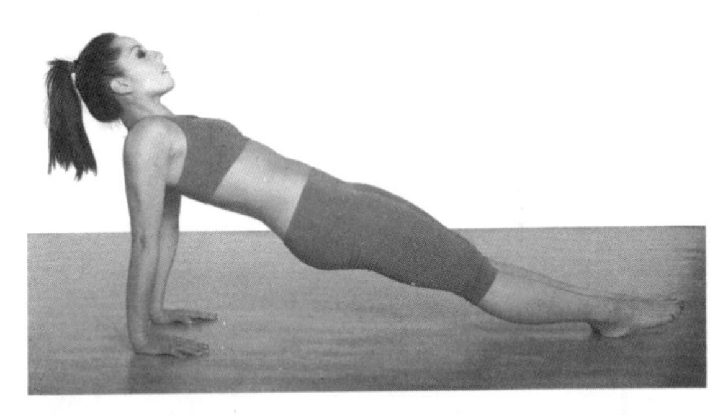

2

CROCODILE PLANK

1 Starting from arm plank position (page 90), with your hands together under your chest, lower down so you're in the bottom of a push-up position (page 79) only supported by your hands and feet. Keep your midsection tight.

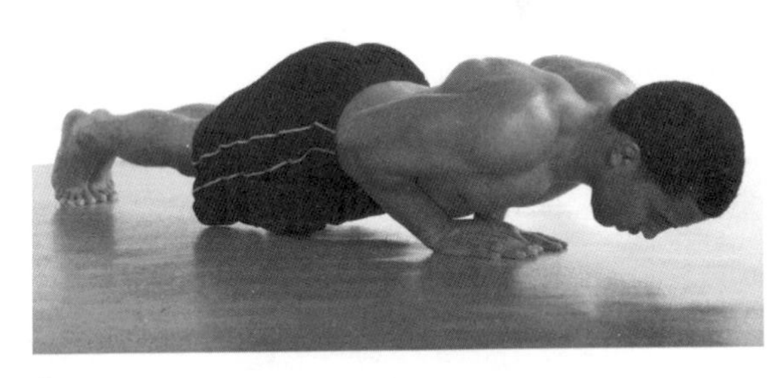

1

WALL SIT

From a standing position, lean back against a wall. Walk your feet out away from you and bend your knees 90 degrees, pressing your back flat against the wall. Hold this position.

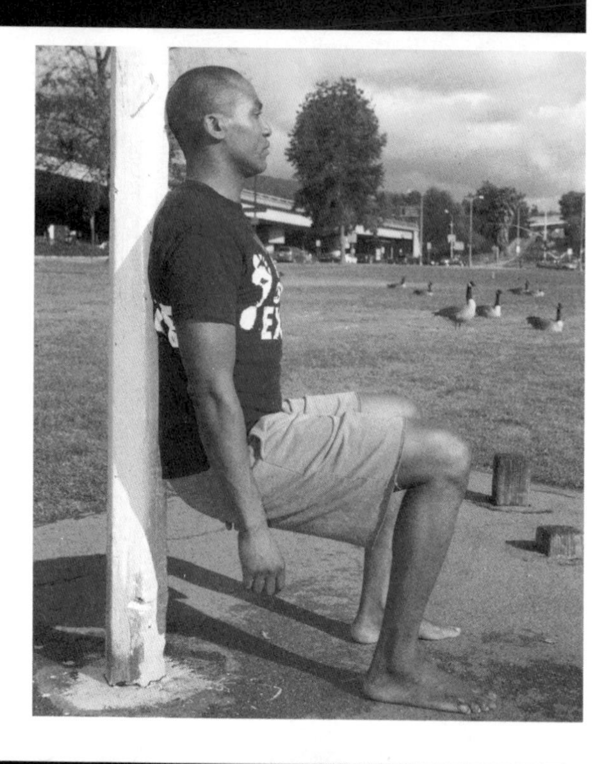

HUNTER-GATHERER (PRIMAL) SQUAT

This is a sitting position common in cultures that don't rely on chairs. It's a very deep squat where your butt is close to your heels. It'll help to reverse some of the damage caused to our bodies by the Western habit of sitting in chairs all the time.

Start from a standing position and sink down into a very deep squat. Keep your heels flat and get your butt as close to your heels as possible. Rest in this position, with a rounded back and relaxed posture.

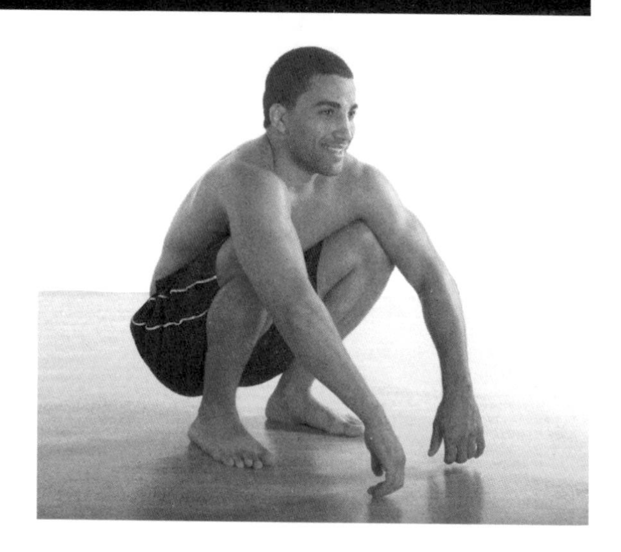

SQUAT HOLD

Follow the instructions for the basic Squat (page 74), but hold at the bottom of the position for the required amount of time.

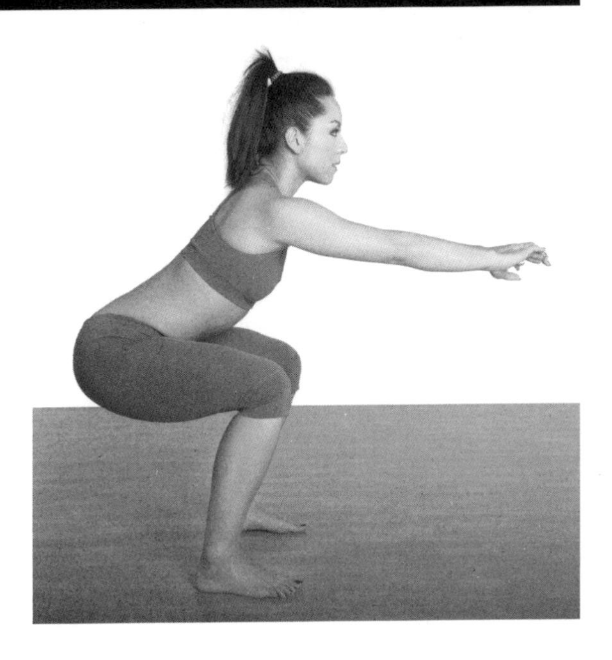

Locomotive Work and Play

Animal Walks

Crawling is a fundamental movement pattern we develop at the earliest opportunity, usually around six months to 1 year old, but it's often neglected once we leave childhood. The process of learning to crawl is actually pretty complex. Babies need to coordinate the movement of their arms and legs, and develop strength in their upper body and legs to support their weight.

Moving on all fours (or quadrupedal movement) is natural, and as adults we can relearn the fun and simplicity of crawling around while gaining proficiency in full-body integrative movement, agility and coordination, and improving cardiovascular and muscular endurance.

Be sure to move slowly during these moves, with good body control and coordination. These exercises strengthen the whole body and improve joint integrity.

Climbs

Children love to climb, and it's usually one movement pattern they master even before standing or walking. Part of this is to develop upper body and core strength. Climbing typically begins once the child has the ability to crawl, initially by crawling over objects, then climbing onto objects such as furniture. They eventually up the complexity by climbing backward down steep gradients such as stairs.

BEAR CRAWL

1 Start in a crouched position and drop onto all fours with your hands directly under your shoulders. Fully extend your arms, then rise up onto the balls of your feet. Make sure your hips are not too high off the ground and keep your body fairly low.

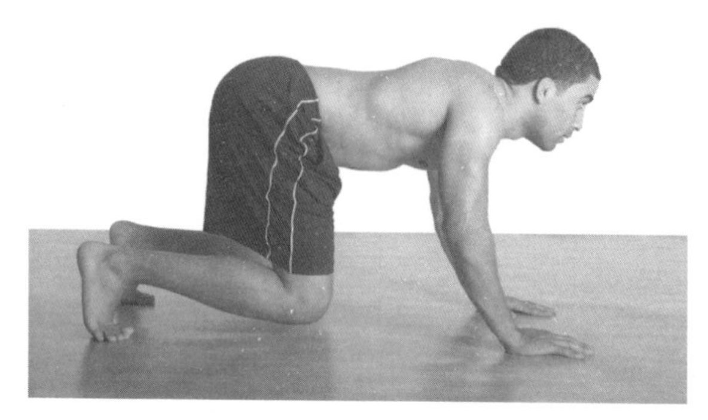

1

2–3 Stay light and animal-like as you crawl forward on your hands and feet. Keep your knees off the ground but don't pull them in too close to your chest. The movement should be contralateral—that is, moving the opposite arm and leg. For example, start moving the right hand, then the left leg, left hand then the right leg to move forward.

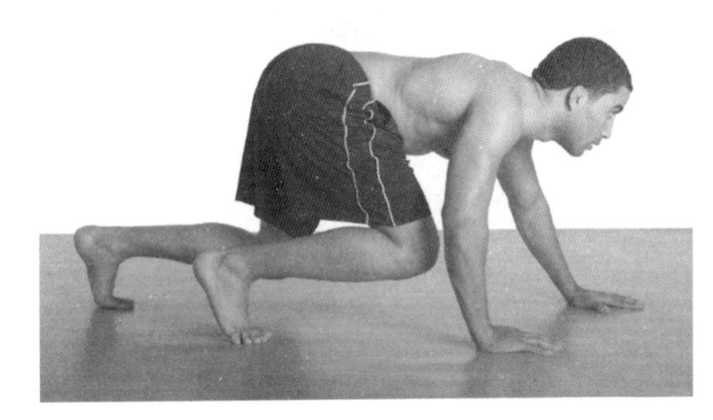

2

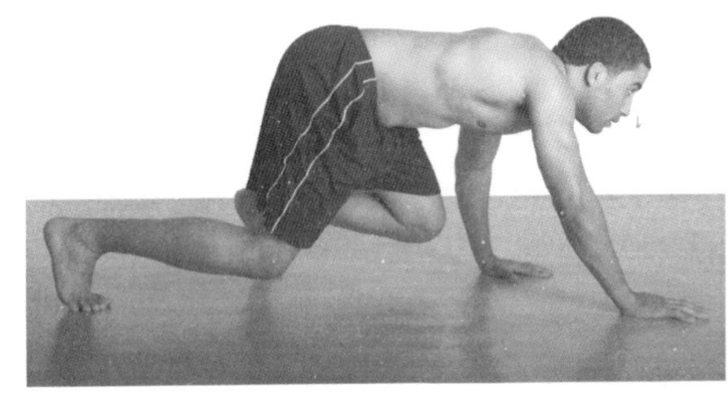

3

VARIATIONS: Crawl backward, sideways, to the left/right and diagonally. Crawl up stairs and down stairs. Crawl uphill and downhill. To add resistance, crawl while holding dumbbells or rocks.

UP STAIRS/UPHILL CLIMB VARIATION: Start in Bear Crawl position and climb up stairs on all fours using the bear crawl technique. Avoid using your knees. You can also do this going down stairs or downhill.

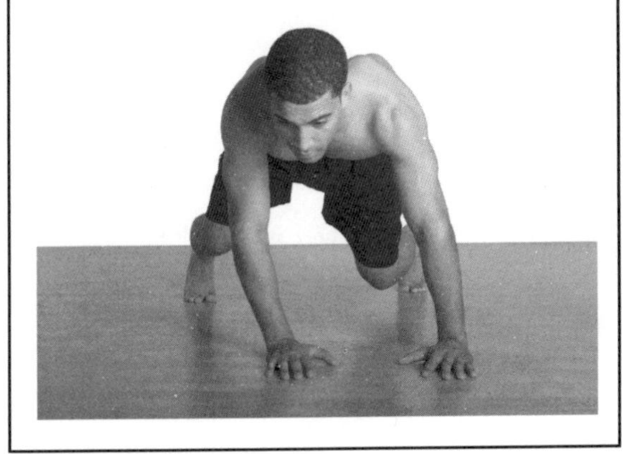

CRAB WALK

1 From a low squat position, place your hands behind your body and lift your hips so your bottom is off the ground. Keep your palms and feet flat on the ground, finding a position that is comfortable for your wrists.

2 Start walking forward. The movement should be contralateral, that is, moving the opposite arm and leg. For example, start moving the right leg, then the left hand, left leg then the right hand to move forward.

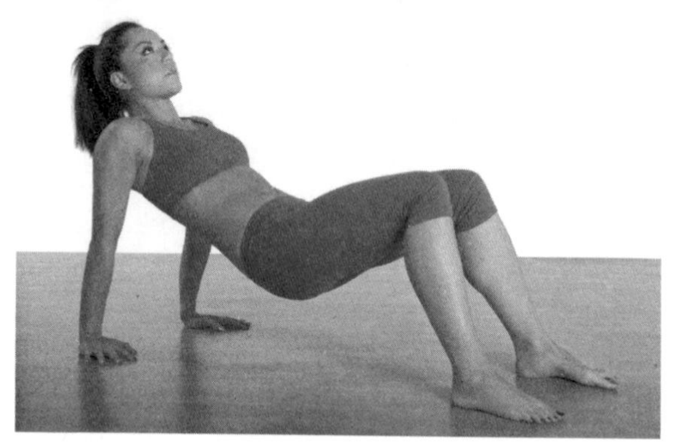

1

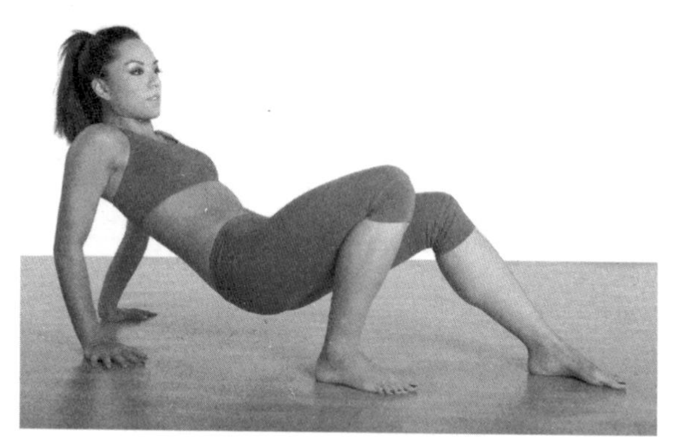

2

VARIATIONS: Walk in all directions: left, right, forward and backward.

STAIRS/DOWNHILL CLIMB VARIATION: Start in Crab Walk position and climb down stairs on all fours using the crab walk technique, taking one step at a time.

CAT WALK

1 From a crouched position, drop onto all fours with your hands directly under your shoulders and arms extended, then rise up onto the balls of your feet. Your knees should be directly under your hips, and arms in line with your shoulders. Ensure your hips are not too high off the ground and keep your body fairly low. Make sure your knees are not pulling in too close to your chest when crawling.

2–3 Stay light and cat-like as you crawl forward on your hands and feet, keeping a strong arch in your back. Keep your back arched throughout the crawl. The movement should be contralateral, moving the opposite arm and leg (e.g., start moving the right hand, then the left leg, left hand then the right leg to move forward). This move is always slow and controlled with small, deliberate movements. Stay in a very straight line.

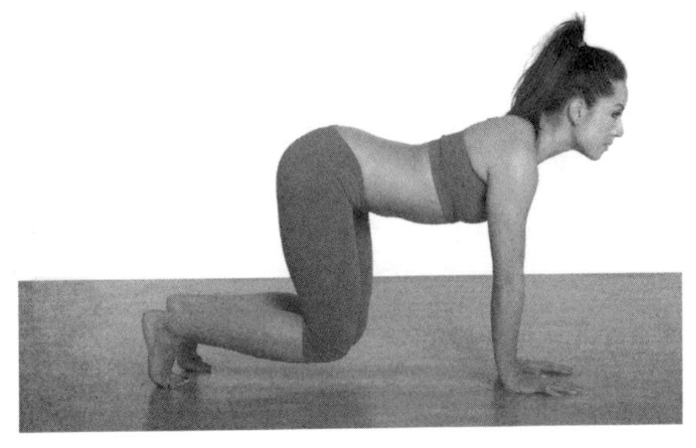

1

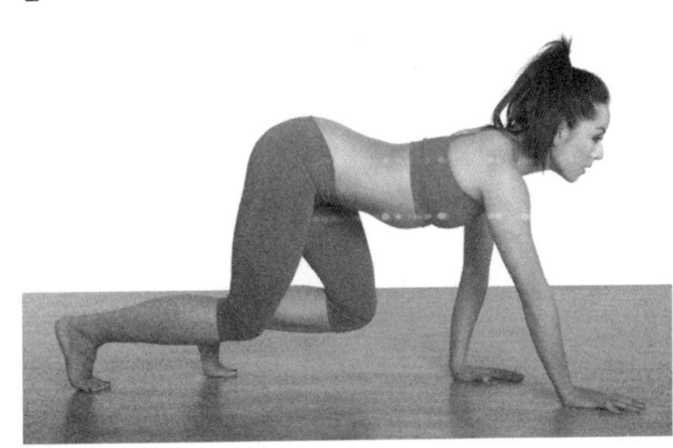

2

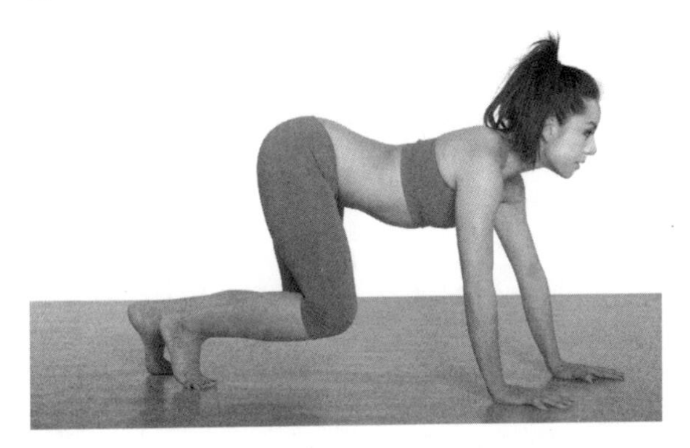

3

SALAMANDER PRESS-UP

1 Start in a low squat position.

2–3 Walk your hands out in front of your body and twist your body as you press down with your right hand in line with your head, left hand in line with your chest.

Keep your body close to the ground and return to starting position. Repeat on the opposite side.

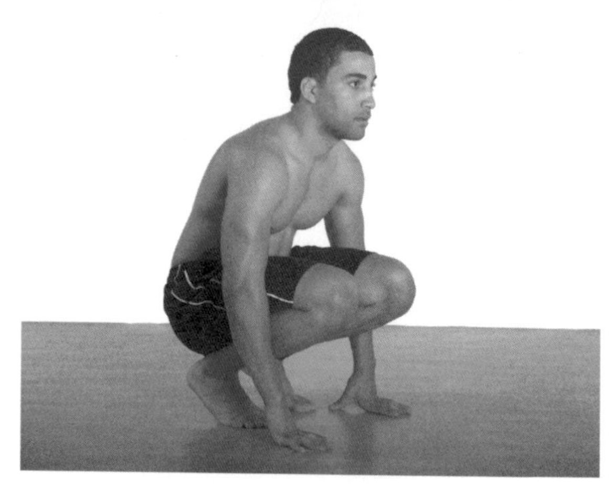

1

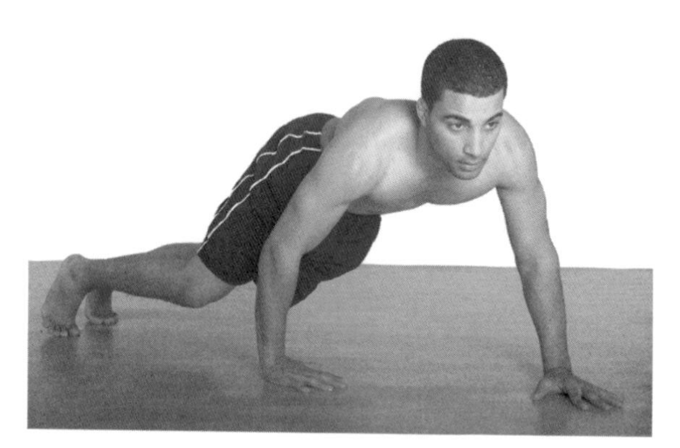

2

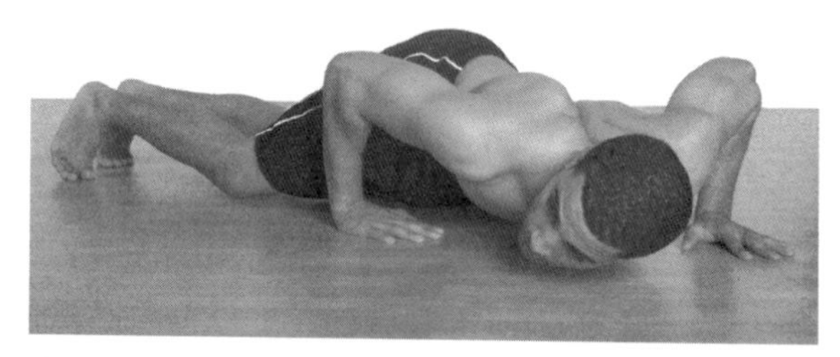

3

RABBIT WALK

1 Start in a low squat position.

2 "Hop" forward onto your arms. Tighten your midsection to keep your knees tucked into your chest. Aim to grab a bit of "air time."

3 Drop to your feet with control.

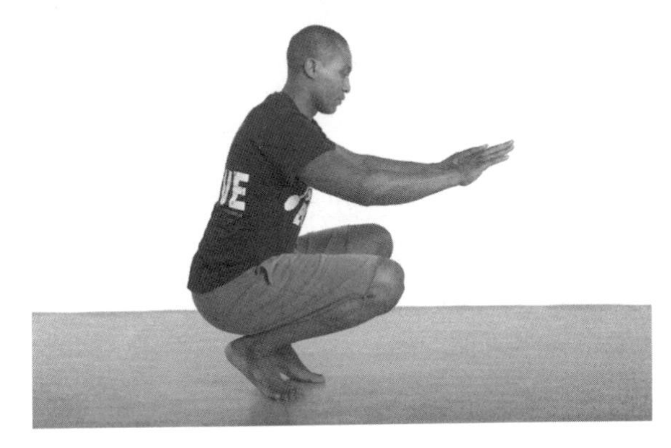

1

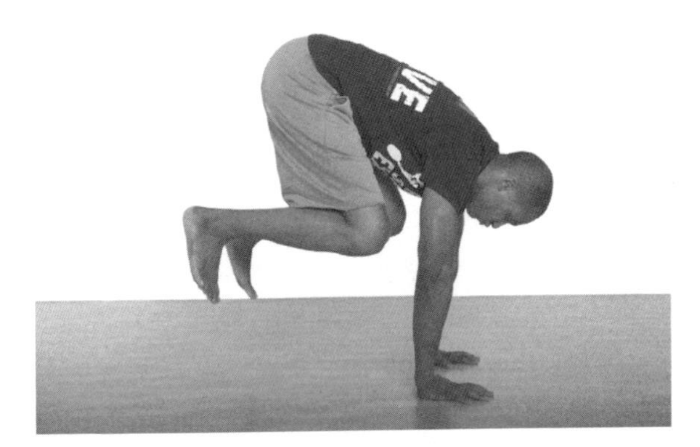

2

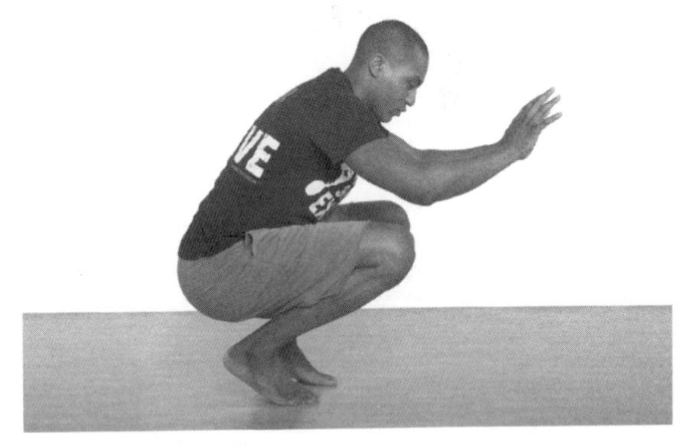

3

CROCODILE WALK

This improves strength and muscular endurance and requires full core activation, coordination and control. It's more difficult than it looks!

1 From arm plank position (page 90), lower down so you're in the bottom of a push-up position (page 79). Get as low as possible, with only your palms and toes touching the ground. Your hands should be in line with your chest. Keep your midsection tight.

2 Shuffle one hand and foot forward at a time, staying as low as possible. Try not to bounce.

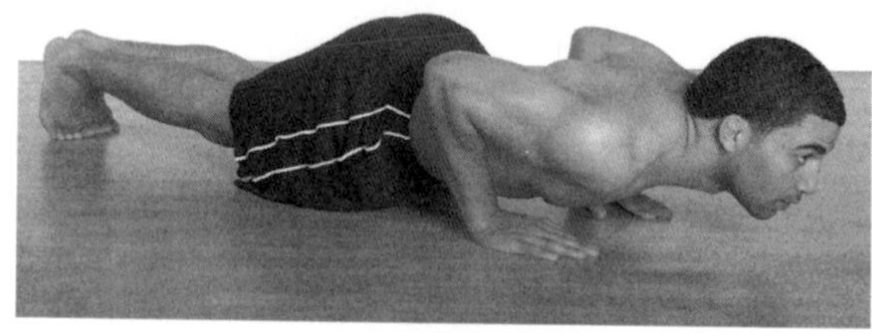

1

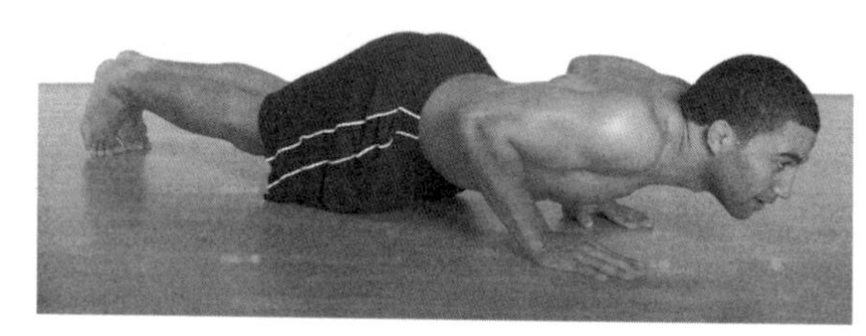

2

DUCK WALK

1 Start in a low squat position, with your arms resting at your sides.

2–3 Walk forward while maintaining the low squat position and an upright torso. You may need to lean forward to stay balanced. Make sure you keep your forward foot flat with your weight on the heel. Stay on the ball of your foot with the opposite foot.

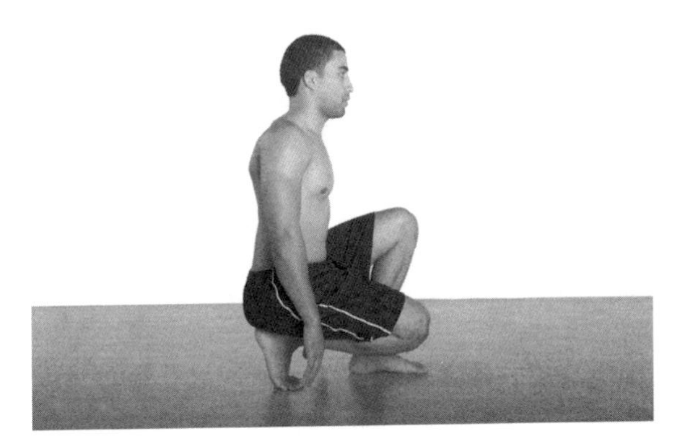

1

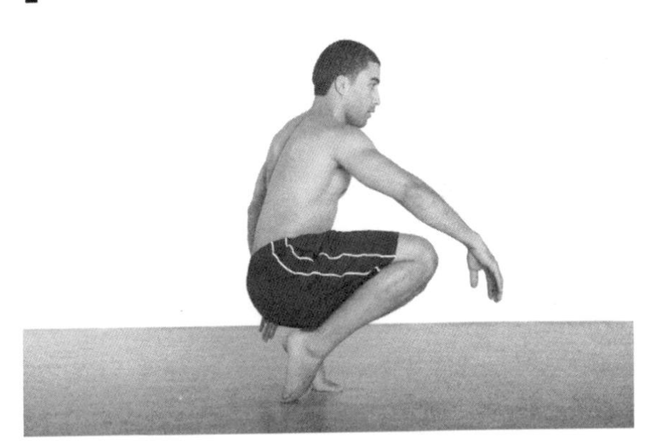

2

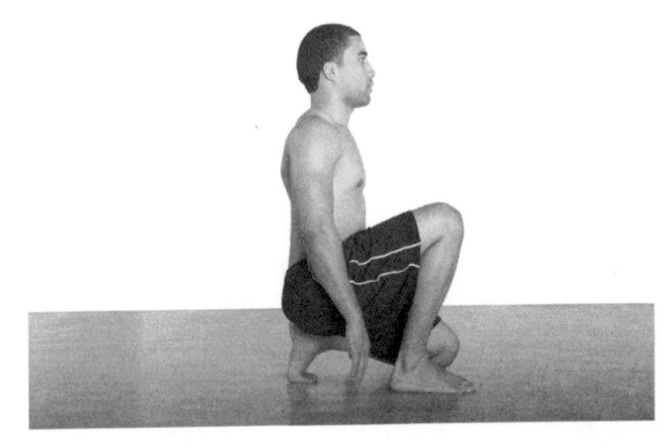

3

TODDLER CLIMB

1 Kneel in front of a chair, sofa, bench or raised platform of similar "sitting" height with your knees shoulder-width apart. Make sure the platform can fully support your body weight. Place both hands flat on the edge of the platform shoulder-width apart, with your arms fully extended and elbows slightly bent.

2 Keeping your hands in place, raise your knees slightly off the ground, keeping your knees bent and shoulder-width apart and balancing on the balls of your feet.

3–4 Keep your core tight and use slow and controlled movement to place your right hand on the floor. Once the right hand is in place, place your left hand down on the floor.

Reverse the movement by slowly raising your left hand until it's back on the platform, then raising your right hand back to the platform. Aim for very soft and quiet movements to ensure low impact on the joints. Continue.

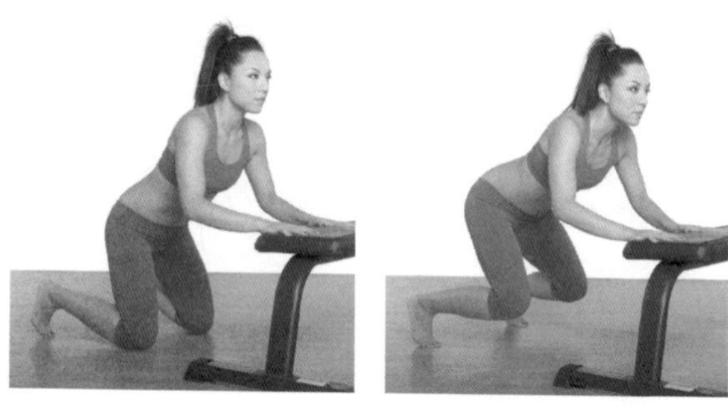

1 **2**

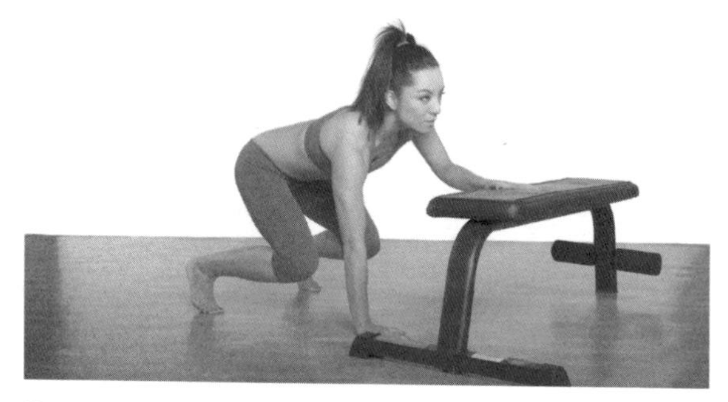

3

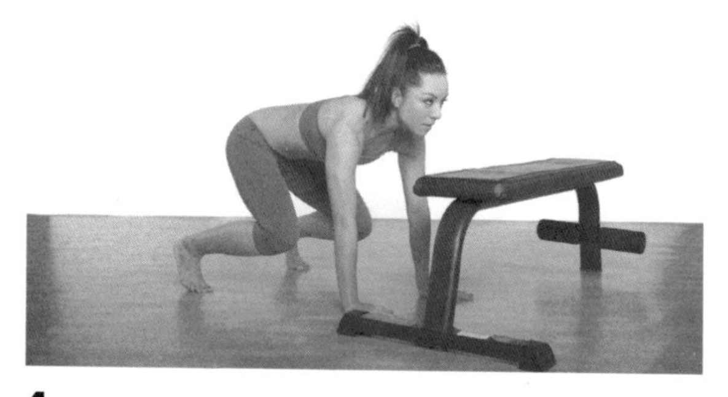

4

VARIATIONS: To increase instability, keep your hands and feet much closer together. To really challenge the core, go for half- or quarter-speed movement. You can also perform the movement at greater speed but still maintain control, or you can change the height of platform.

TODDLER TRAVERSE

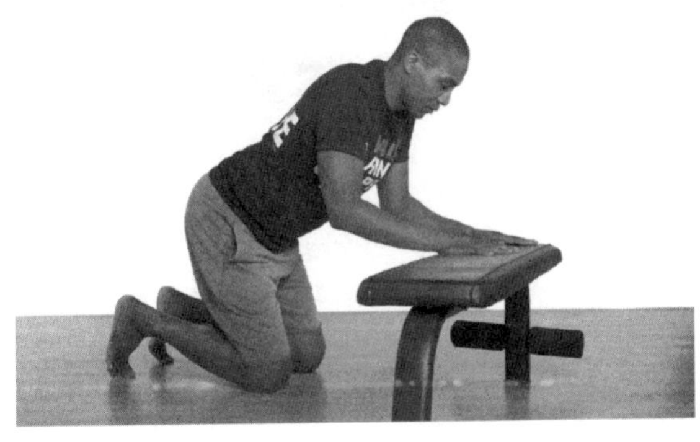

1

1. Kneel in front of a chair, sofa, bench or raised platform of similar "sitting" height with your knees shoulder-width apart. Make sure the platform can fully support your body weight. Place both hands flat on the edge of the platform shoulder-width apart, with your arms fully extended and elbows slightly bent.

2. Keeping your hands in place, raise your knees slightly off the ground, keeping your knees bent and shoulder-width apart and balancing on the balls of your feet.

3. Moving from left to right, "walk" your right hand a couple of inches to the right and follow with your right foot. Then "walk" your left hand a couple of inches to the right and follow with your left foot.

   Continue and reverse direction as required.

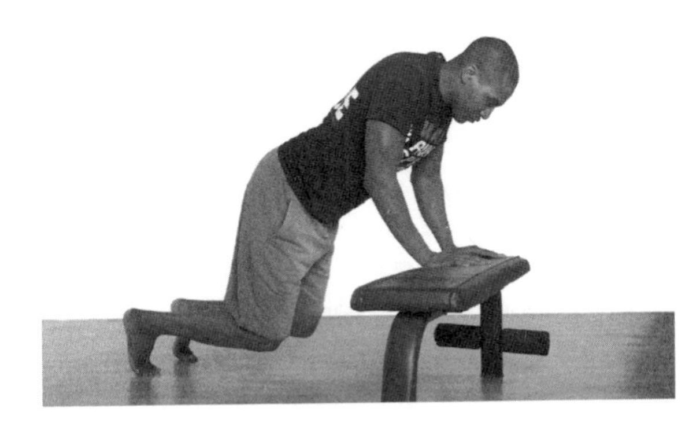

2

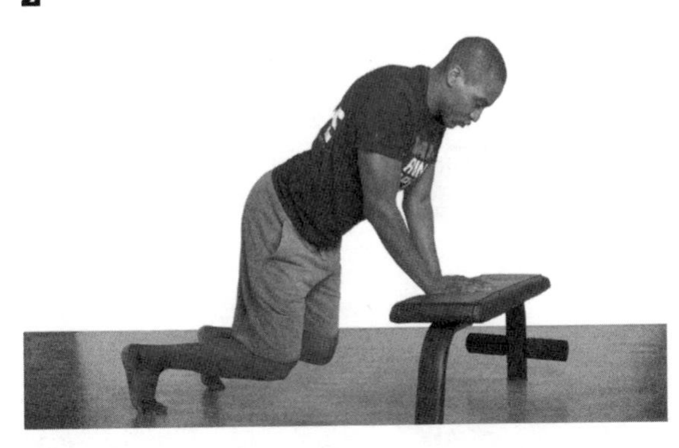

3

VARIATIONS: Try this movement with your hand and foot moving at the same time, or try it with straightened legs (similar to a plank position).

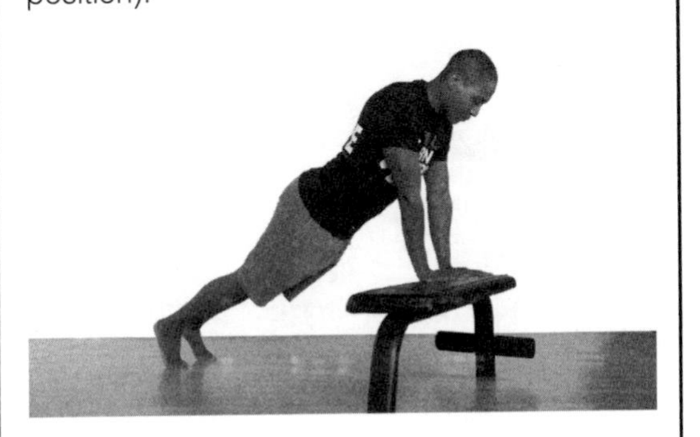

Hangs & Pull-Ups

DEAD HANG

This is the starting position for the pull-up. Beginners will find that the ability to hold onto the bar is difficult. The limiting factor is often forearm and grip strength. The Dead Hang will help build strength in those muscles to help you ultimately perform a full pull-up. However, if you can't perform a Dead Hang at all, do an Inverted Hang (page 111) instead until your strength builds. If you don't have access to a pull-up bar, use a climbing frame or tree branch. A tree branch is more challenging because the texture of the bark and the increased circumference make it more difficult to grip.

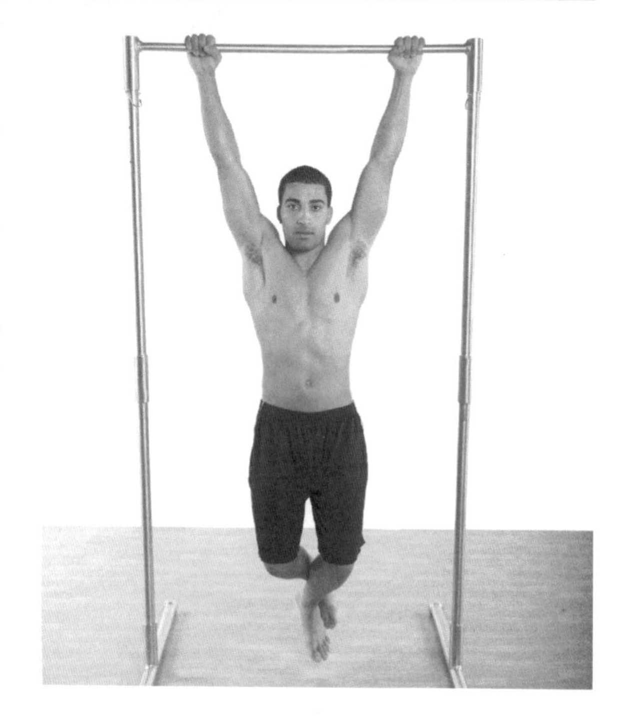

Hang from a pull-up bar with your hands in line with your shoulders. Keep your lower body relaxed and don't let your feet touch the ground. See how long you can hang for.

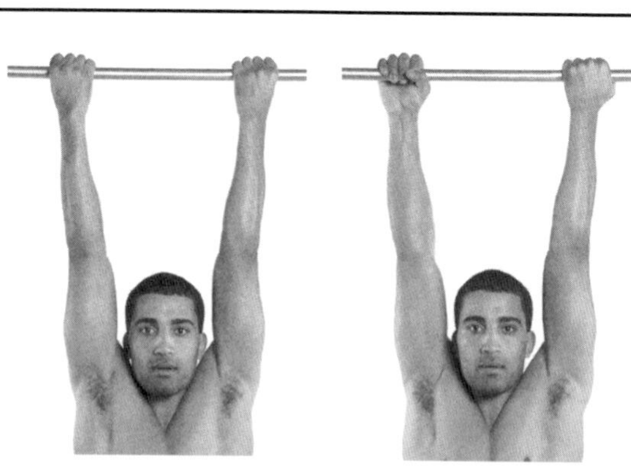

GRIP VARIATIONS: You can also use the chin-up grip (underhand) or mixed grip (one hand underhand, one hand overhand).

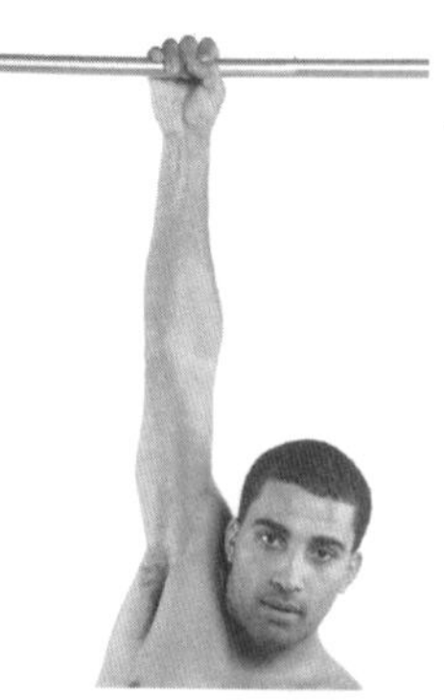

SINGLE-ARM VARIATION: Hang with one arm as long as possible.

CHIN-OVER

Using an underhand grip, get your chin above the bar and hang there as long as you can. Keep your body as still as possible but try to stay relaxed.

When you can no longer hold this position, lower slowly into a dead hang and release with a soft landing.

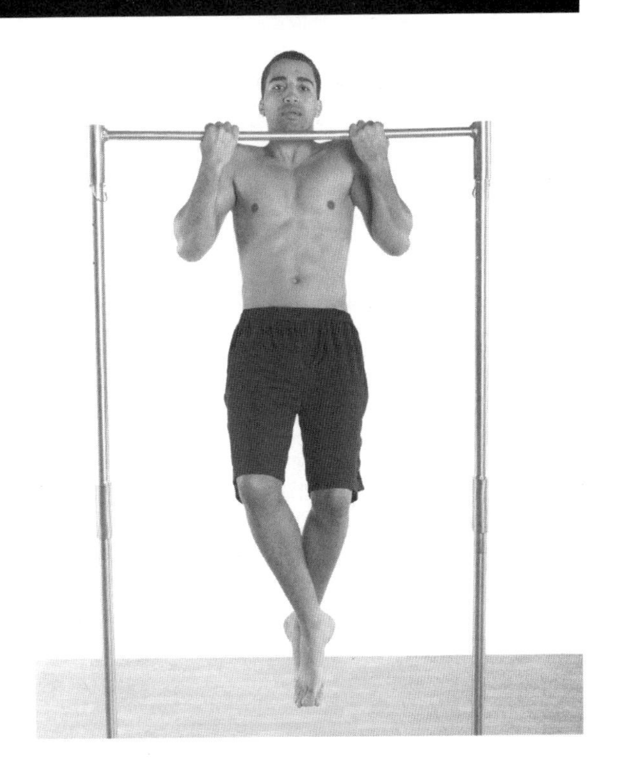

PULL-UP

Pull-ups are a total-body exercise, with the back, torso and even the legs working to achieve the movement. Good grip strength is essential for pull-up performance, so try to avoid using gloves or wrist straps. They may make the job slightly easier but the best way to improve forearm strength is to avoid the use of supports.

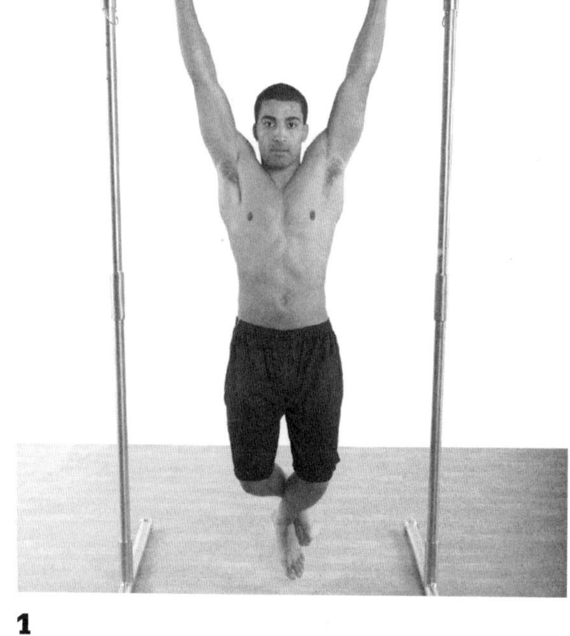

1

1 Hang from a pull-up bar with your hands in line with your shoulders or slightly wider. Use an overhead grip and keep your shoulders active and packed into their sockets.

2 Minimizing movement in the body (don't swing), pull yourself up toward the bar and get your chin over it. Aim to increase the range of the pull by getting your chest closer to the bar.

Lower yourself with control until you return to starting position. Pause and repeat, avoiding swinging your legs or using momentum to bounce back up.

MODIFICATIONS: If you're unable to lift your body weight, there are ways to reduce your body weight to make the exercise easier. You could use a strong helper to support some of your weight, or you can hang a strong resistance band over the bar and stand or kneel in it to provide extra leverage. Over time reduce the amount of support as you get stronger.

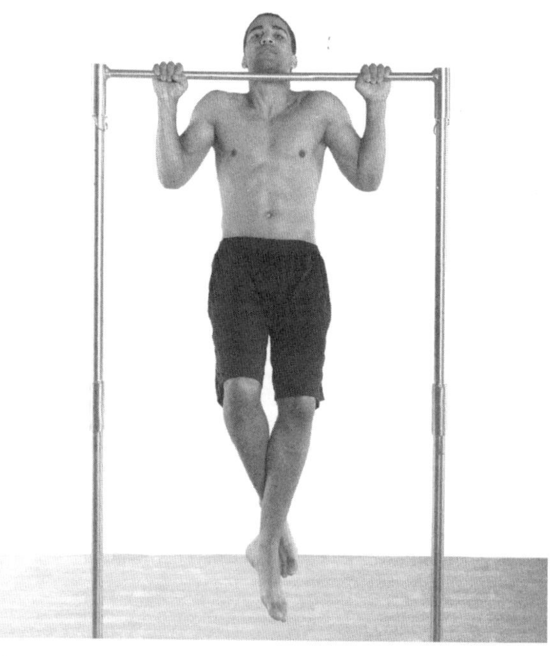

2

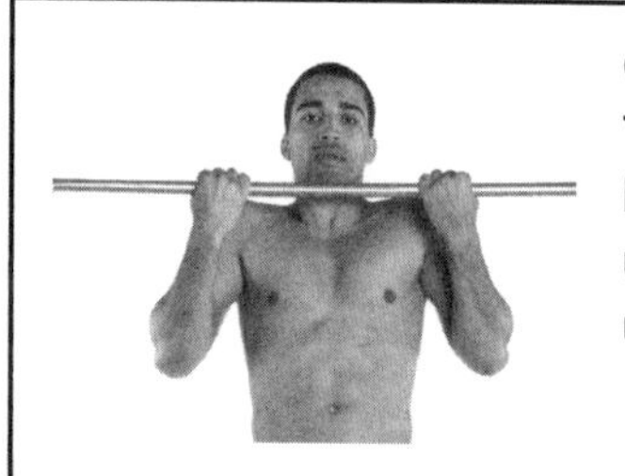

CHIN-UP VARIATION: Perform a pull-up using an underhand grip.

JUMPING PULL-UP

1–3 Jump up from the floor or a raised platform (such as a box, if necessary) and get your chin over the bar using an overhand grip. Most of the power comes from the legs for this move. Be sure you can't reach the floor or raised platform from a dead hang position.

Lower yourself slowly and repeat.

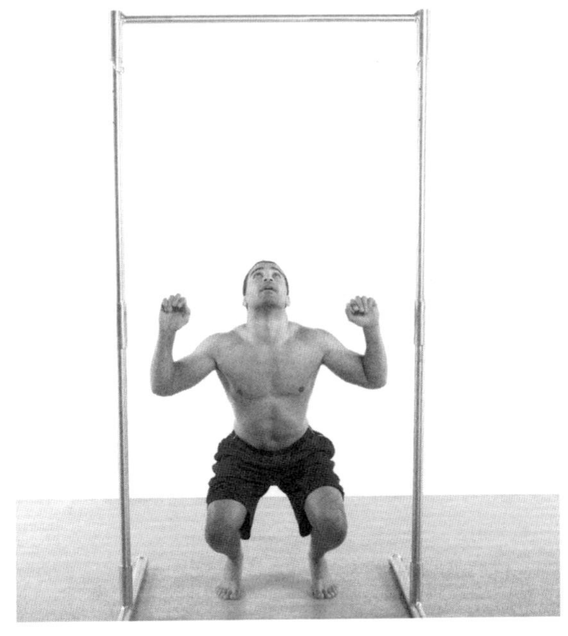

1

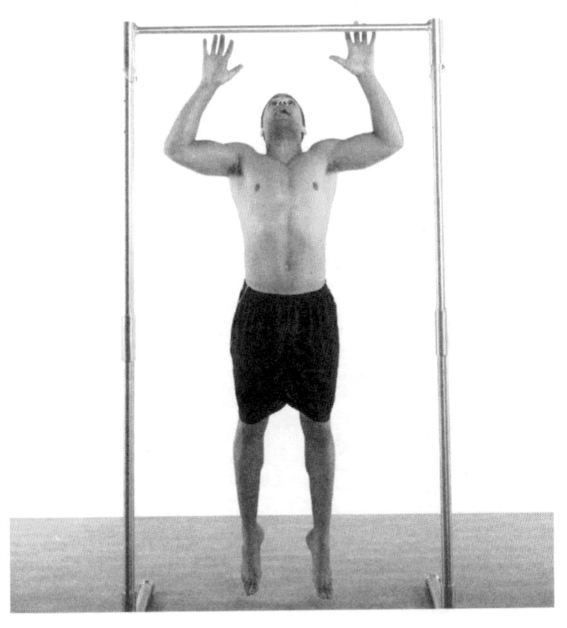

2

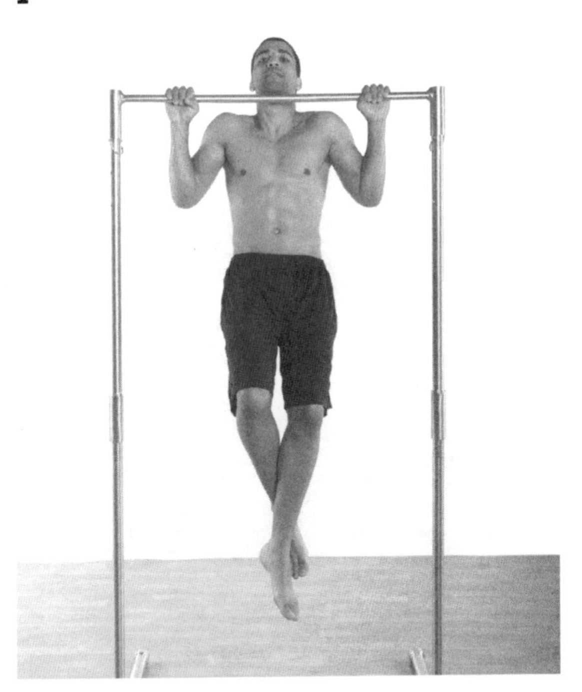

3

MUSCLE-UP

1 Hang from a pull-up bar with your hands in line with your shoulders or slightly wider. Use an overhead grip and keep your shoulders active and packed into their sockets.

2 Pull up explosively, as quickly as possible, getting your chest to the height of the bar. Bend at the elbows, get your chest over the bar, and rotate your palms.

3 Straighten your arms and push your chest up until your hips touch the bar.

Reverse the movement with control.

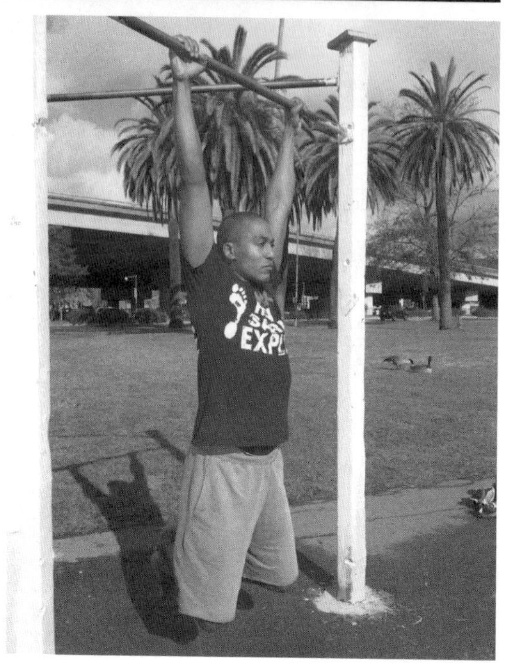

1

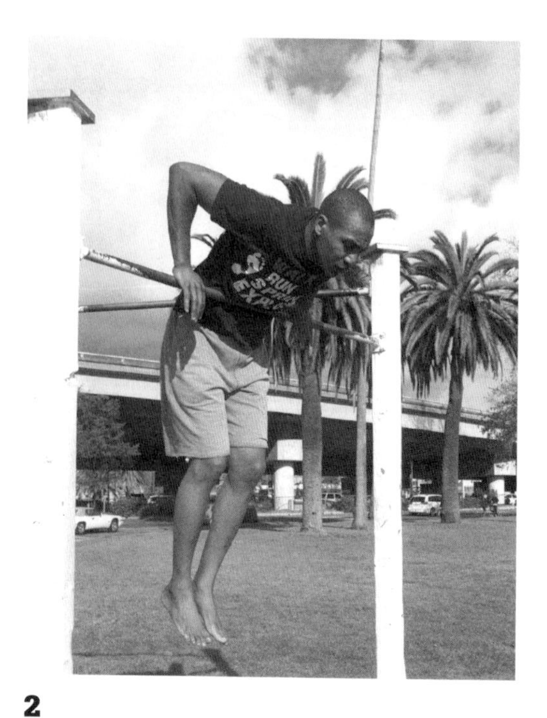

2

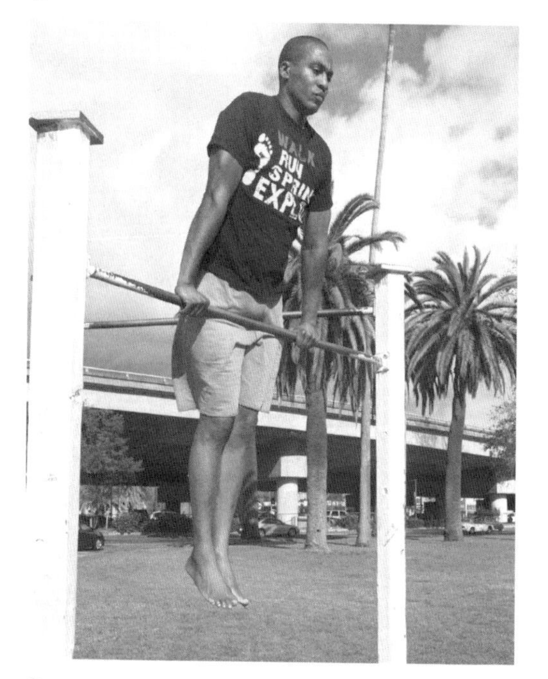

3

POWER PULL-UP

1 Hang from a pull-up bar with your hands in line with shoulders or slightly wider. Use an overhead grip and keep your shoulders active and packed into their sockets.

2–3 Pull yourself up as quickly as possible to get your chest to the height of the bar. At the top of the pull, briefly release your hands from the bar. Catch the bar on the way down.

Lower yourself with control until you return to starting position. Pause and repeat.

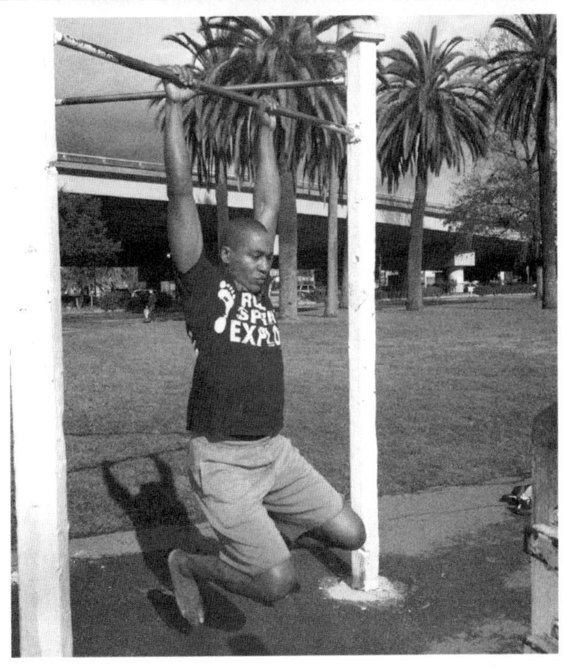

1

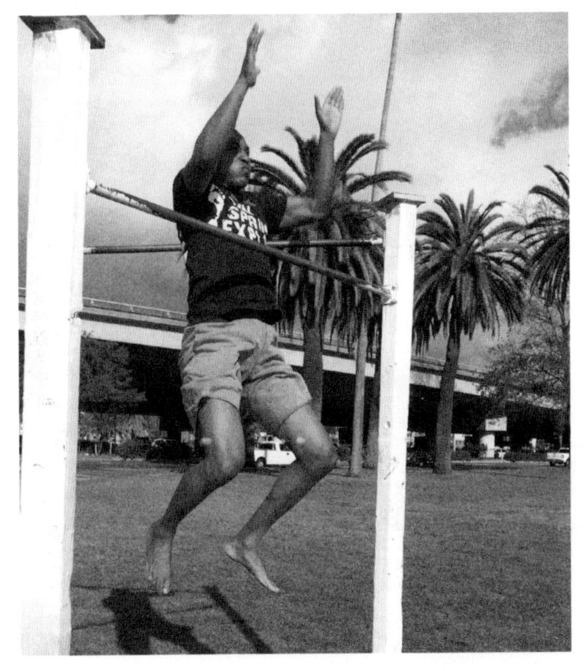

2

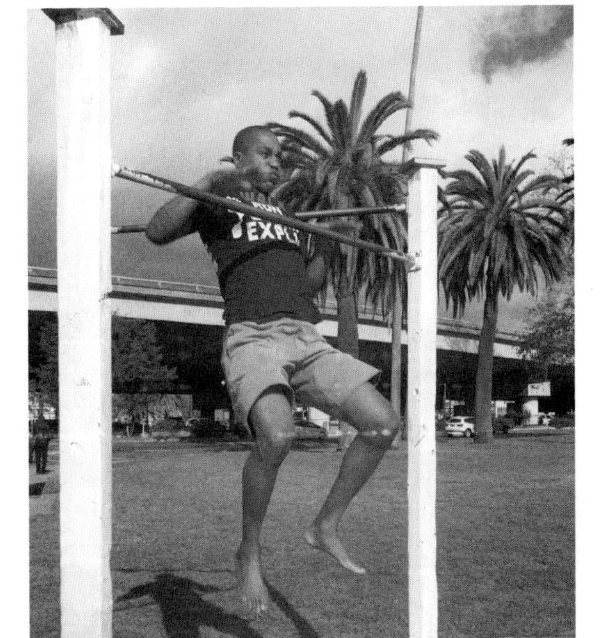

3

TOES-TO-BAR

1 Hang from a pull-up bar in Dead Hang position (page 104). Palms can be underhand or overhand.

2 Bend your knees, brace your midsection and bring your toes up to touch the bar.

Minimize momentum (don't swing) and use slow, controlled movement to lower your legs back down to starting position. Aim to hold onto the bar throughout the movement.

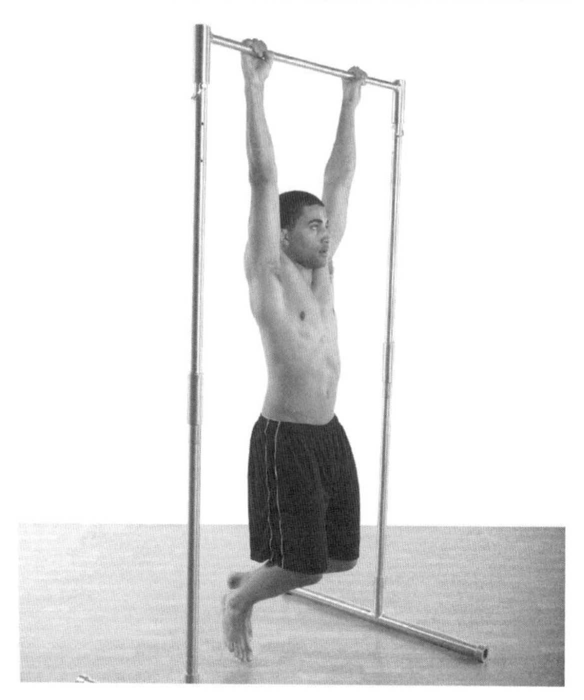

1

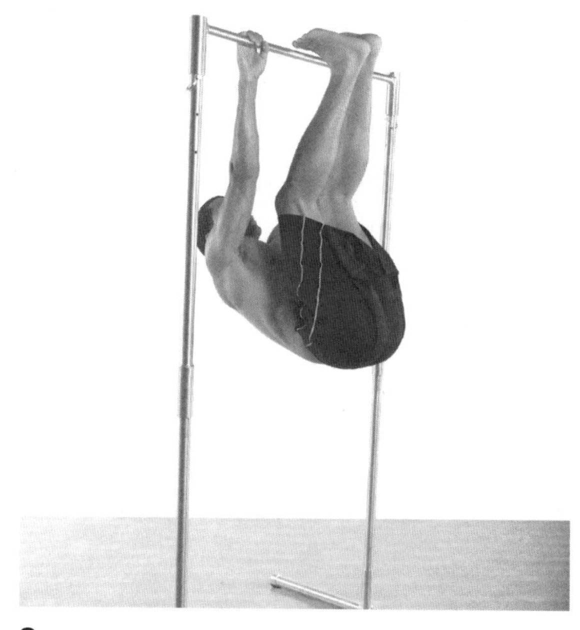

2

INVERTED HANG

If you're not quite ready to do a Dead Hang (page 104), this is a good beginning exercise to build strength in those muscles.

1 Position a pull-up bar about 3 feet off the ground. Get under the bar and grasp it using an under- or overhand grip.

2 Keeping your whole body in a straight line from heels to shoulders, head and body in alignment, bring your hips off the ground. Your feet should be together and up on your heels. Hold this position without allowing your body to sag.

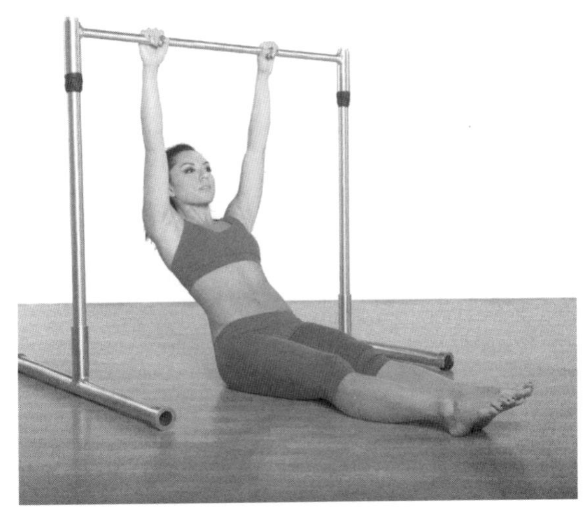

1

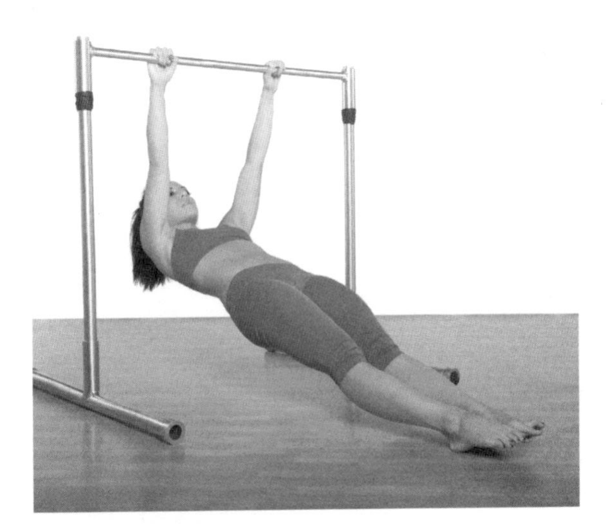

2

INVERTED ROW

1 Hang from a pull-up bar in Dead Hang position (page 104) with your legs and body straight. Palms can be underhand or overhand.

2 Using your feet as a pivot point with heels touching the ground, pull your chest up to the bar. Avoid any sagging in the body and maintain a strong core.

Lower yourself with control until you return to starting position. Pause and repeat.

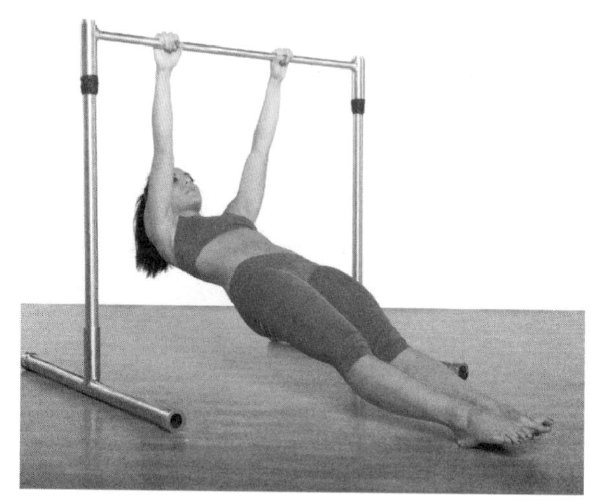

1

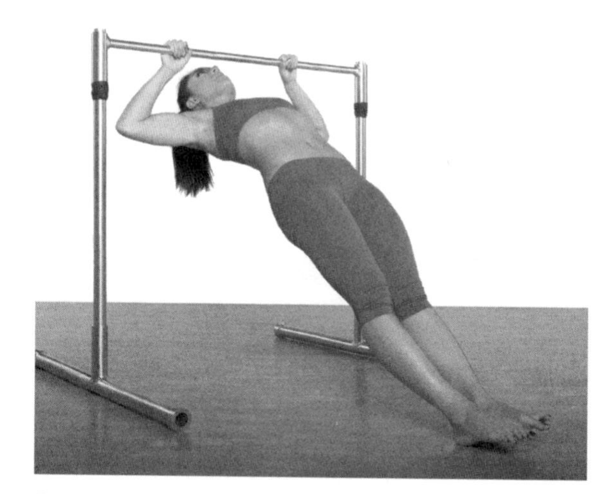

2

Jumping

An expression of power, a jump requires speed and strength to execute effectively. Any air time gained is the satisfaction of beating gravity even for a brief moment. The landing is more important than the absolute height gained or distance jumped and needs to be focused on first to prevent jarring the joints and sustaining injury. Always land on the balls of your feet. A great way to improve landing ability is through jumping rope, emphasizing landing softly on the balls of your feet.

BUNNY HOP

1 Crouch down into a low squat with your feet about shoulder-width apart and hands clasped behind your head. Raise your heels off the ground.

2 Hop on the balls of both feet for very short distances at a very low height. This move can be performed forward, backward, left, right and in place.

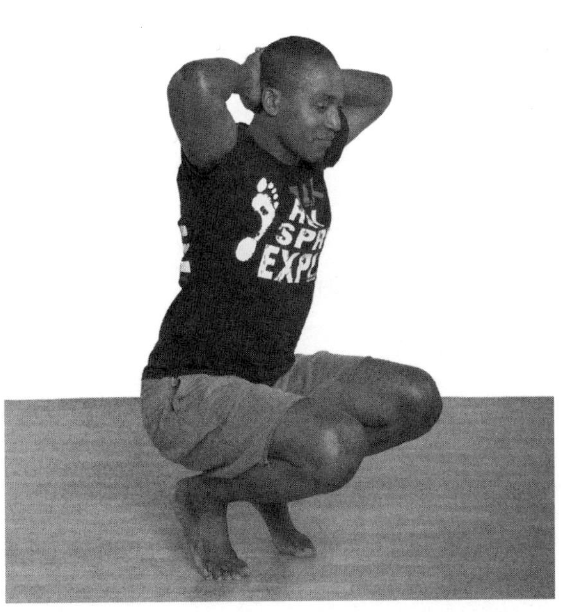

1

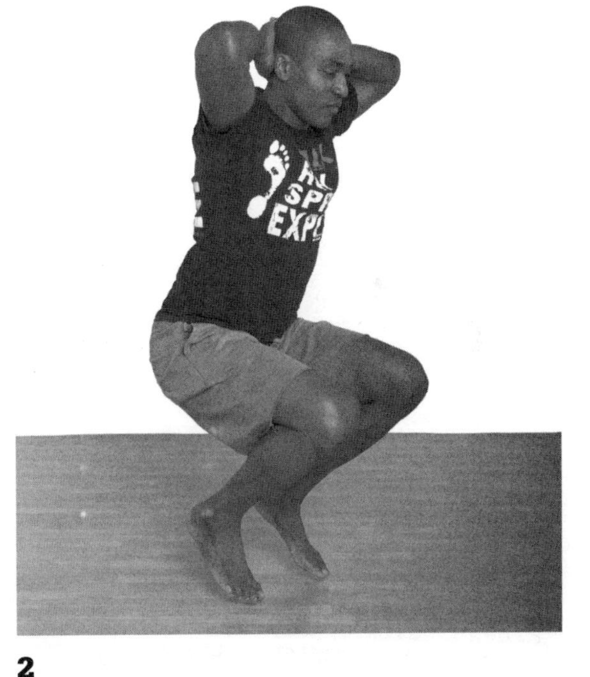

2

TUCK JUMP

1 Stand tall with your feet shoulder-width apart and your arms hanging at your sides.

2–3 Lower to a quarter-squat, then jump and bring your knees up to your chest. Aim for maximum height.

Land softly and with control, like a cat, on the balls of your feet.

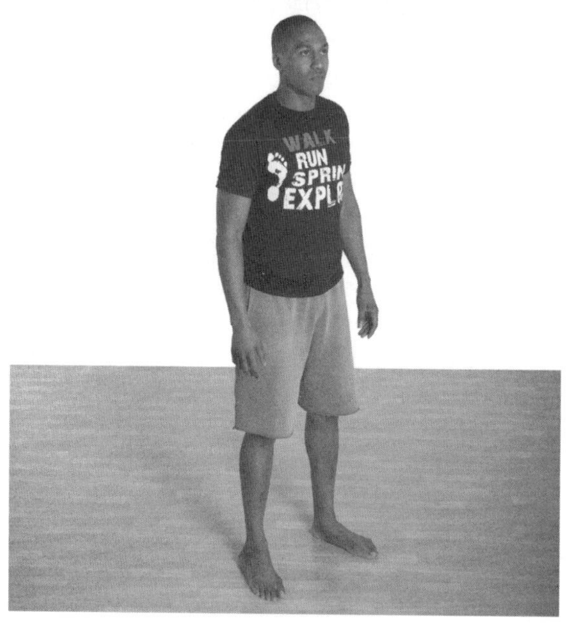

1

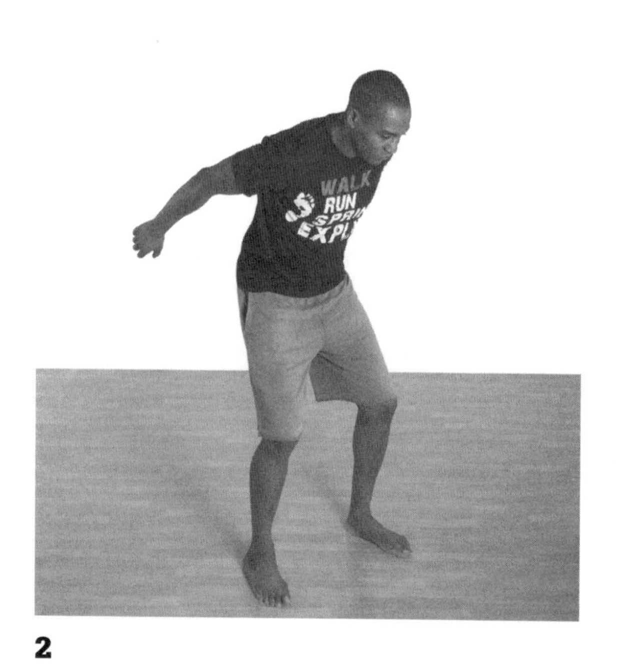

2

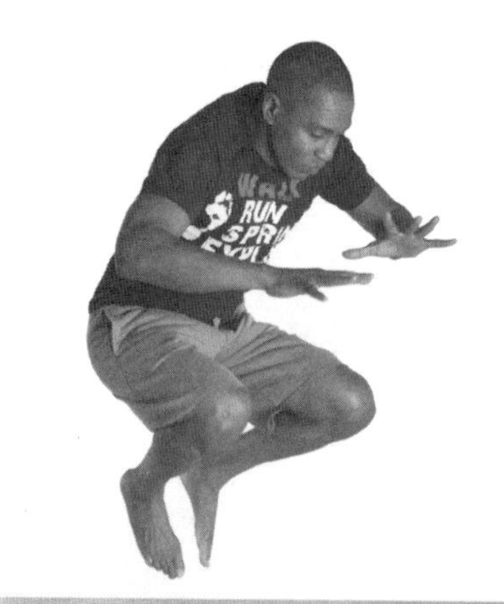

3

SQUAT JUMP

1 Stand tall with your feet shoulder-width apart and your arms hanging at your sides.

2–3 Lower to a quarter-squat, then jump as high as you can, keeping your whole body as straight as possible. Aim for maximum height.

Land softly and with control, like a cat, on the balls of your feet.

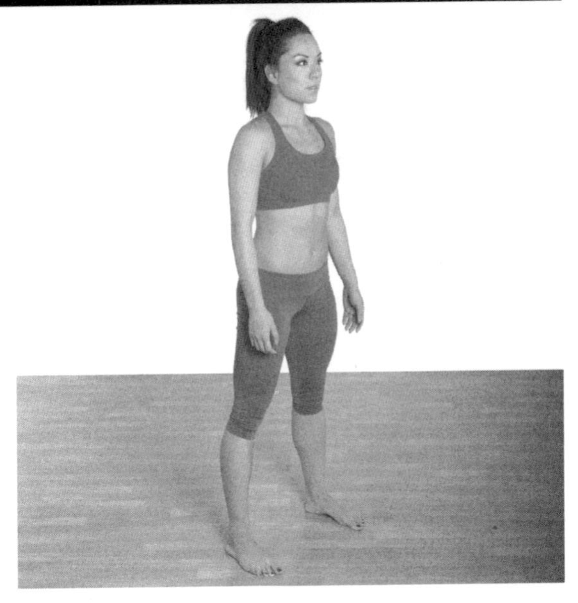

1

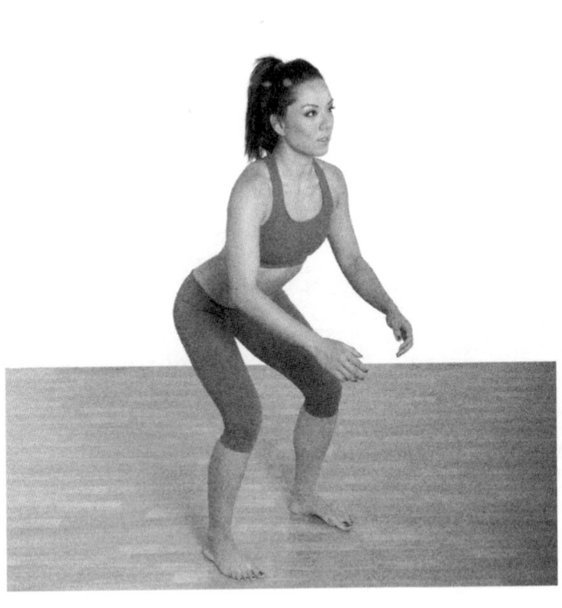

2

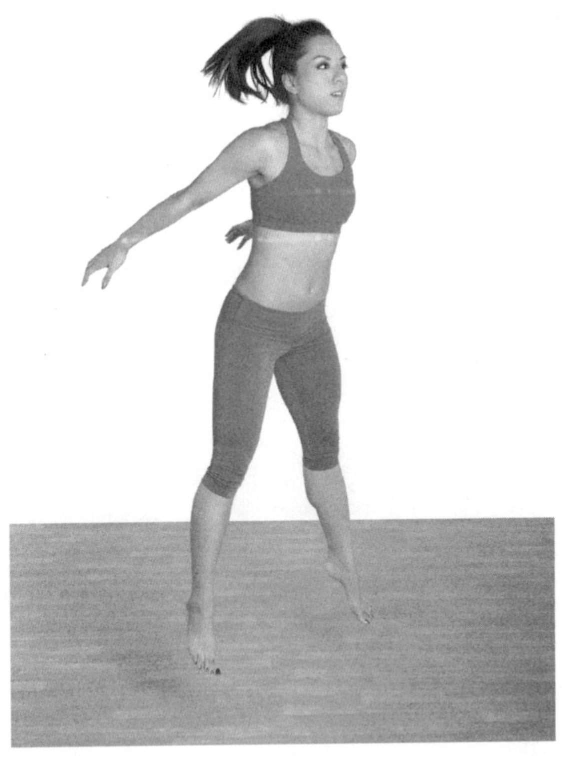

3

KANGAROO JUMP

1 Stand tall with your feet shoulder-width apart and your arms hanging at your sides.

2–4 Swing your arms behind you to generate power, and long jump as far as you can. Land softly and with control on both feet.

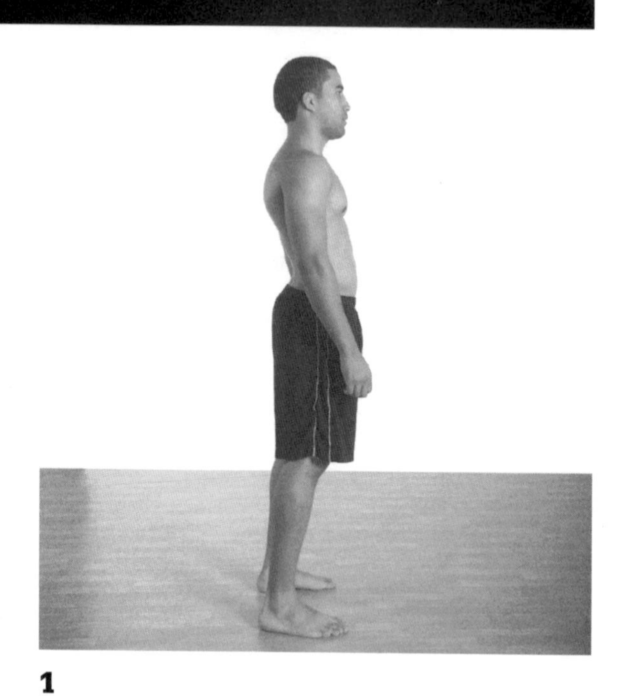

1

2

3

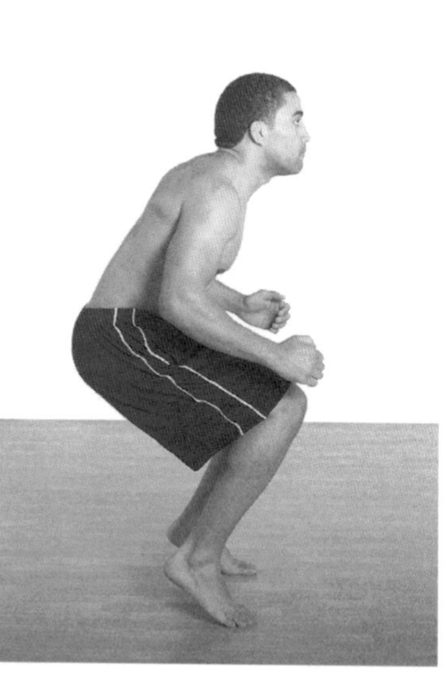

4

JUMP ROPE (SINGLE-UNDER)

This is the jump that immediately comes to mind when someone says "jumping rope." Maintain your balance and time your jumps based on the speed of the rope. As you progress, focus on being "light on your feet" by jumping and landing in a controlled manner. Breathe in a slow and rhythmic manner—make sure you don't hold your breath!

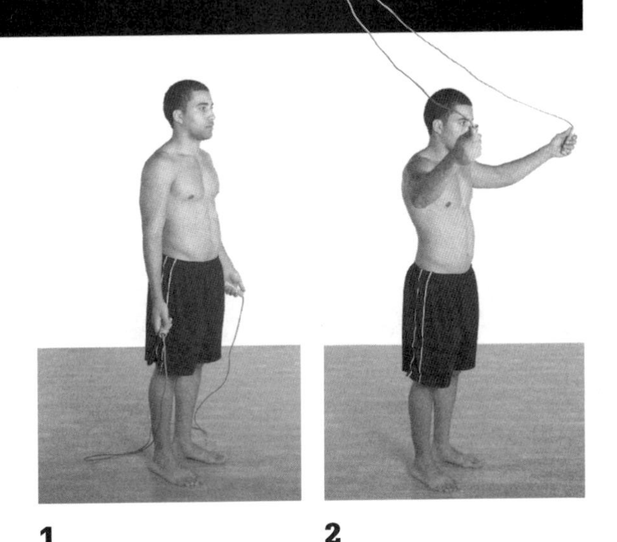

1 2

1 Stand tall with your feet about shoulder-width apart, knees slightly bent, and arms extended along your sides. Throughout the movement your weight should be distributed evenly on the balls of both feet. Start with the rope on the ground behind your feet.

2 Rotate your wrists counterclockwise to swing the rope overhead. The first movement from a dead stop will require more arm and shoulder movement. As you progress on sub-sequent jumps, your arms should remain in a semi-static downward position by the sides of your body. Your hands should rotate counterclockwise in small arcs.

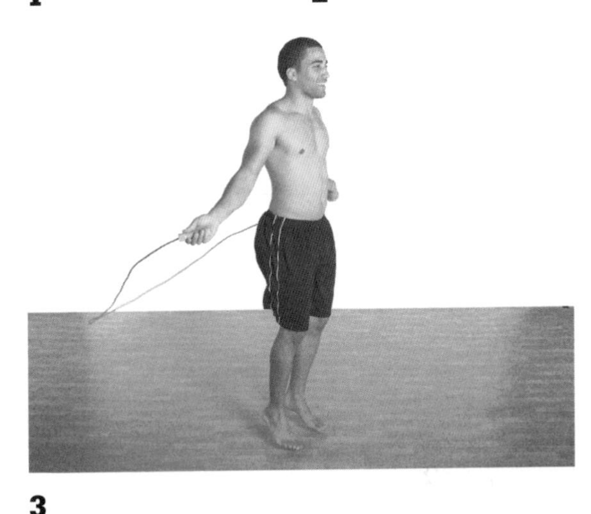

3

3 As the apex of the rope's loop approaches the ground in front of your body and is about 6 inches away from your toes, jump straight up with both feet with just enough clearance for the rope to pass underneath. Keep your legs extended when you jump so they're almost straight.

Land softly on the balls of both feet and bend your knees slightly to cushion the impact while continuing to rotate your wrists and swing the rope in an arc from back to front.

DOUBLE-UNDER VARIATION: In this version the rope travels underneath your body twice per jump. When the rope is about 6 inches away from your toes, jump straight up with both feet a little higher than normal for the rope to pass underneath. Continue your swing quickly while your feet are still off the ground and complete another swing under your feet. Swing speed is the key. You can't do a Double Under without adequate swing speed. If you're having trouble, stick with basic single-unders until you get faster.

Sprinting

Sprinting requires all-out effort. As such it is a high-intensity exercise and one of the most time-efficient workouts you can do. There are many benefits. It naturally produces growth hormone, which offers incredible fat burning. Sprinting burns fat even hours after the workout is over, during the recovery phase. This is based on excess post-exercise oxygen consumption (EPOC), otherwise known as afterburn. Sprinting will strengthen your feet, ankles, calves and legs. It also improves cardio health and strengthens your heart.

CROUCH TO SPRINT

From a low crouched bear crawl position (page 94), spring up and accelerate into a sprint for 30–40 meters. Then decelerate.

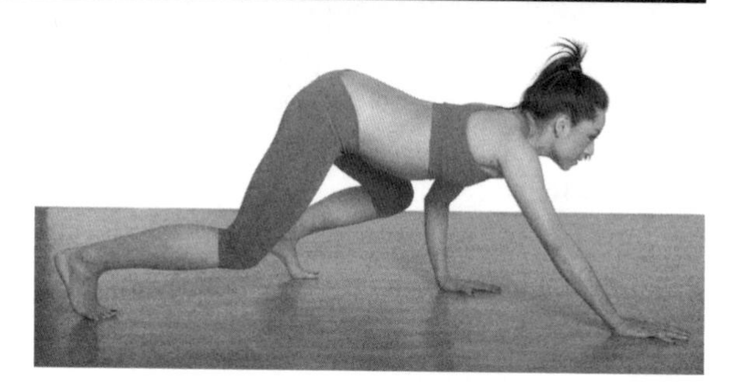

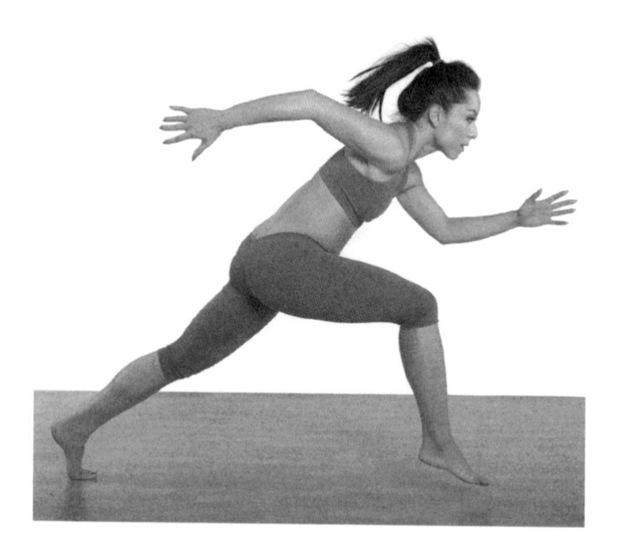

UPPER BODY SPRINT

Start in a standing position with your feet shoulder-width apart. Use your arms and torso only as though you were sprinting as fast as you can. Move your feet and legs as little as possible. Try to minimize hip movement, and keep your upper body facing straight ahead rather than twisting from side to side. Do not hold your breath.

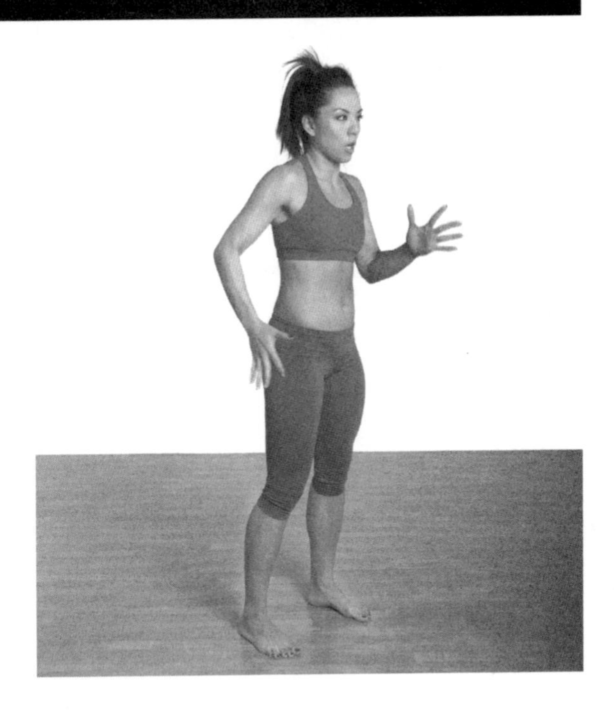

SPRINTING IN PLACE

Simply sprint on the spot, staying very light on your feet.

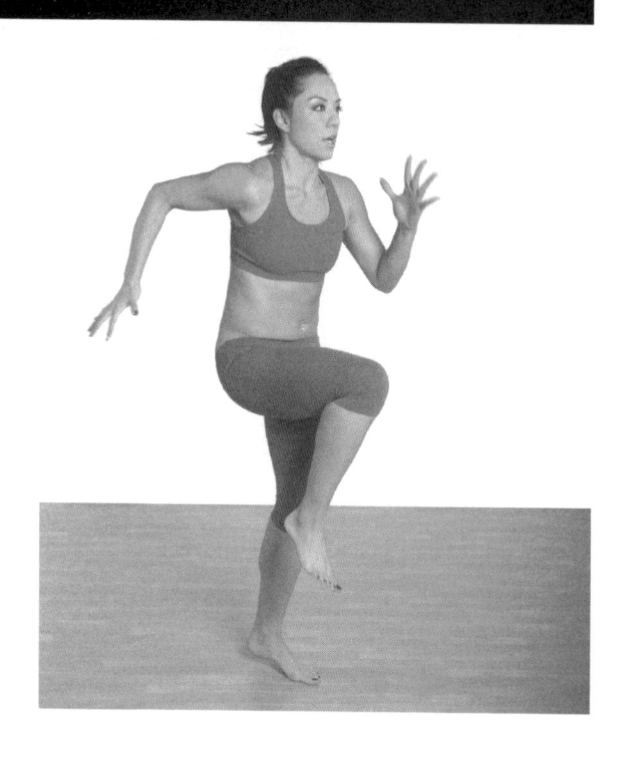

ADVANCED VARIATION: Try to raise your knees in front of you to above hip height.

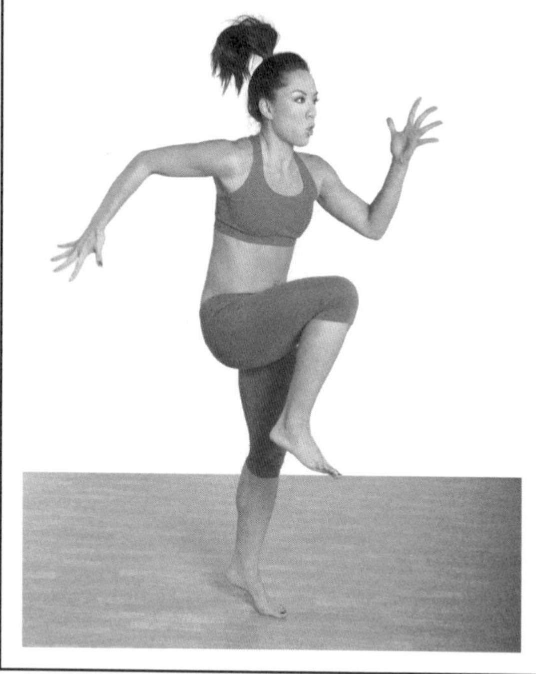

Balance

Balancing is fundamental to any movement we perform. Even when standing, we're maintaining balance even if we're not consciously aware of it. Watching a child learning to stand, you realize the act of balancing itself is the challenge, not the lack of leg or core strength.

With balance we're not only working the often-neglected stabilizer muscles, but also improving joint stability and our internal focus. Balance is also one key skill we lose as we age, so maintaining this is important. It's a use-it-or-lose-it proposition.

FEET-TOGETHER TOE SQUAT

1 Stand tall with your feet together and hands clasped behind your head.

2 Exhale and push up onto the balls of your feet and then onto your toes as high as you can while maintaining balance.

3 Inhale and bend your knees to descend into a squat. Keep your head up in neutral position, and keep your back straight and core tight. Hold briefly at the bottom of the squat.

Slowly return to starting position.

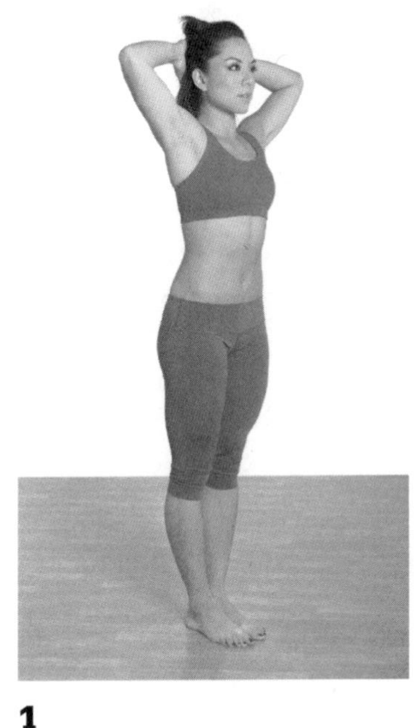

1

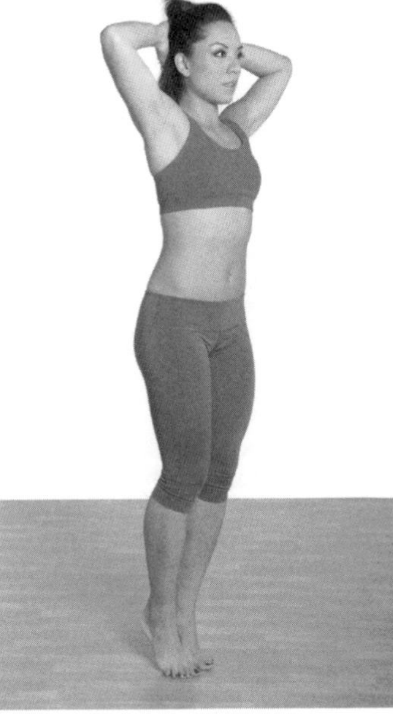

2

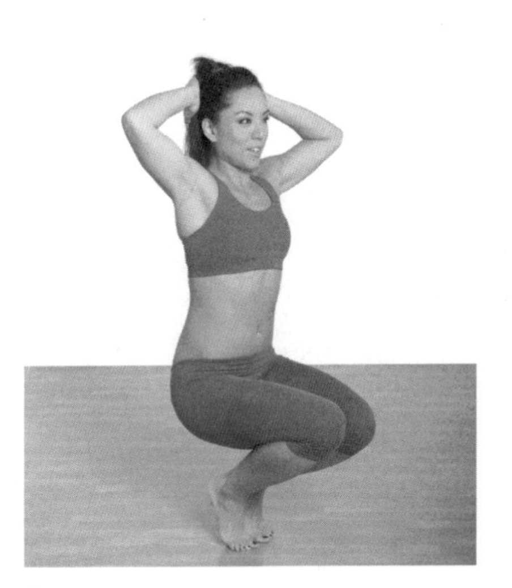

3

TOE STAND

1 Stand tall with your feet together.

2 Rise up and balance on your tiptoes.

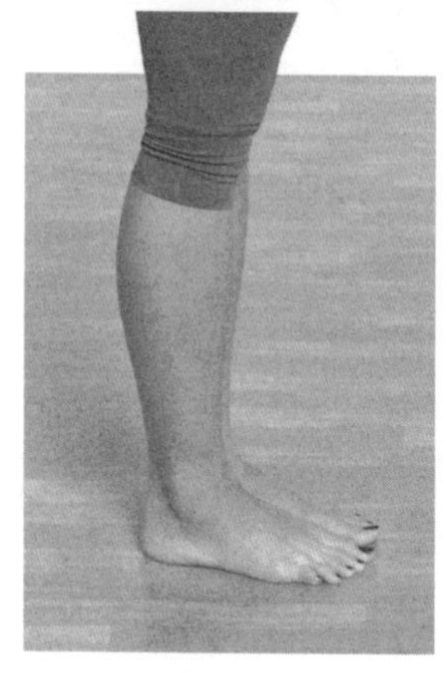

1

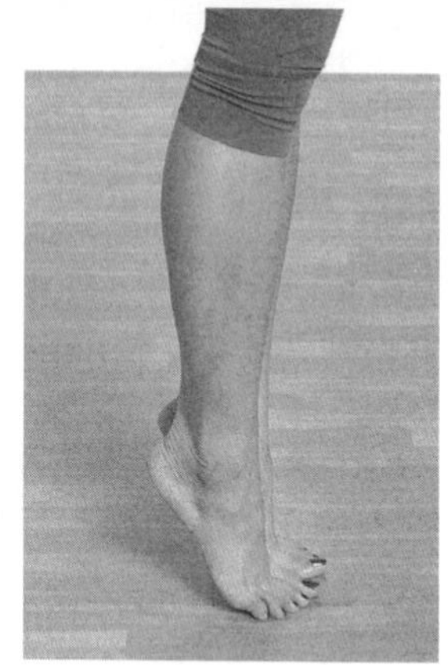

2

HEEL STAND

1 Stand tall with your feet together.

2 Lean back and balance on your heels.

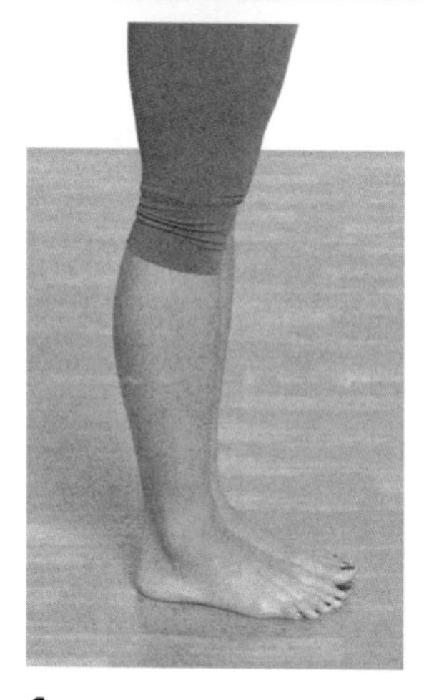

1

2

ONE-LEGGED STAND

1 Stand on one leg and balance for as long as possible.

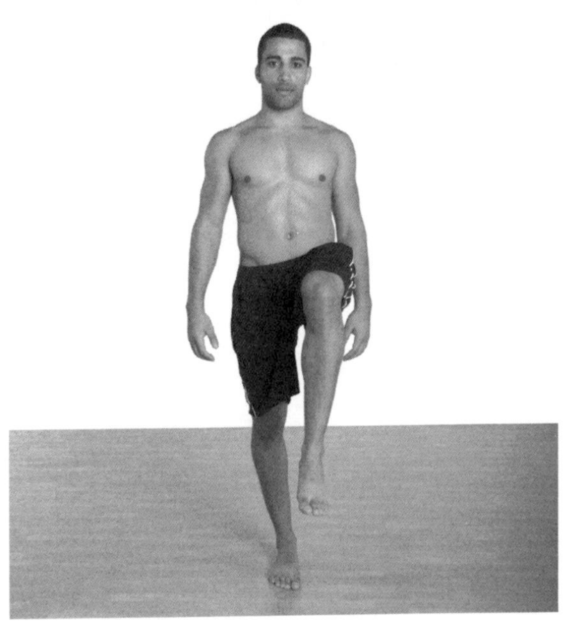

1

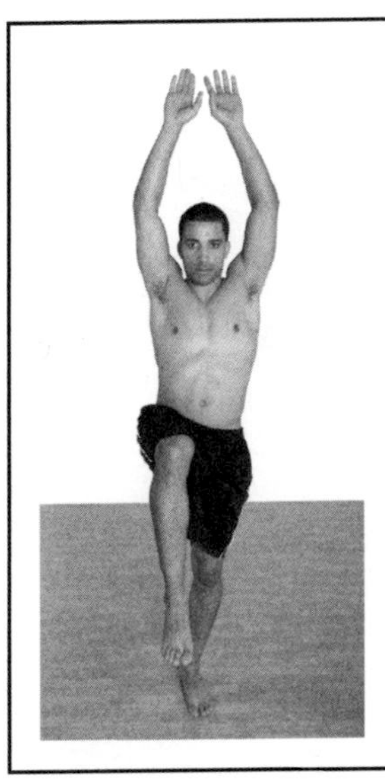

ADVANCED VARIATION: To make it more complicated, close your eyes. For an even more advanced version, place your hands above your head.

SPRINTER'S LUNGE

This move will prepare you for regaining balance after swift and powerful movement.

1 Perform a lunge (page 76) with your right foot forward and left foot back. Hold at the bottom position.

2–3 Jump up explosively, change leg positions midair, and land with your left foot forward and right leg back.

Continue switching. Initially you may hold your hands on your hips to help with balance, but aim to complete this with your arms at the side of your body.

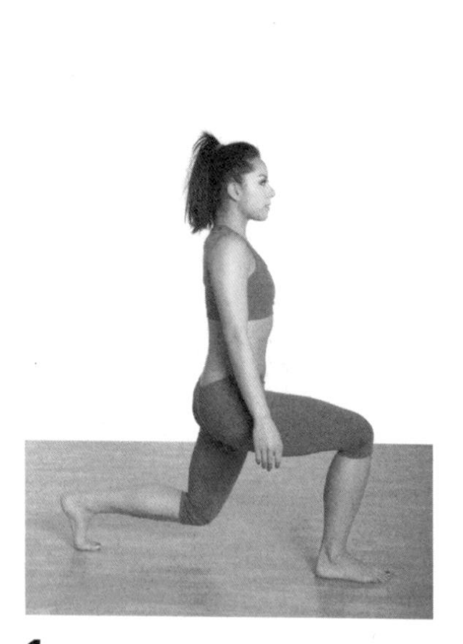

1

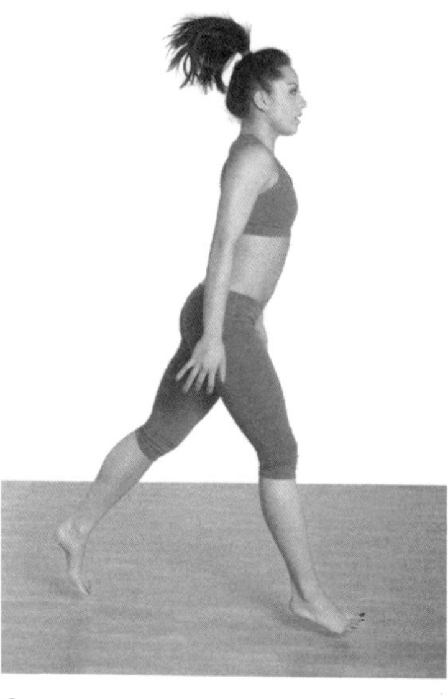

2

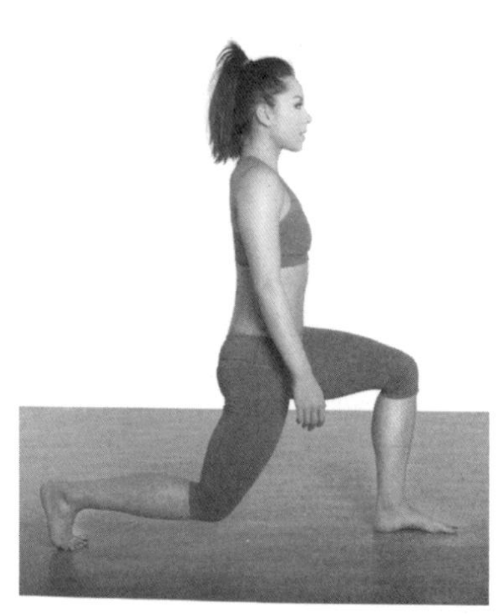

3

Object Work and Play

Be strong to be useful. —Georges Hebert

You've probably seen people lifting weights in the gym but, in practical terms, why would you just lift something just to put it back on the ground? Usually you lift something as a precursor to moving with that object and carrying it to its intended destination. There's a practical reason for having this strength, so our training should incorporate "carrying" too. For these movements, you'll need to either purchase a sandbag or build your own.

Buying or Making Your Own Sandbag

For those athletes who like to get their hands a little dirty, a sandbag can be one of the easiest pieces of equipment to fabricate and use in your workouts. You don't need to spend hundreds of dollars on a fancy dumbbell set or choose what size and weight kettlebell you need to purchase. For as little as a few bucks, you can put together an extremely usable and versatile weight.

Most big hardware stores or nurseries carry suitable bags of sand. Look for a 40-pound version in a tear-resistant bag; these are usually the types of sandbags that are designed for ballast and not what you'd purchase to fill a kid's sandbox. If it comes with a built-in handle, that's fine, but in order to build your grip strength, you'll alternate between using it and not. Your local fire department may also be able to provide some sandbags; they probably won't charge you, so feel free to make a little donation.

Bags of kitty litter or dog food work exceptionally well, provided the bag is strong and the weight is suitable for your workouts. Don't be afraid to use plenty of duct tape to make these weights more durable, but make sure you don't wrap it too tight; a good sandbag will bend, flex and allow the contents to move around a bit inside.

If you'd rather start from scratch and make your own, a heavy garbage bag and some duct tape will be an inelegant yet workable short-term solution and also allow you to select a weight that'll work best for you. Dump as much sand as you'd like into a bag and form it into the rounded rectangular shape of a sandbag. Leave a little room for the sand to shift inside; this'll make your stabilizer muscles work even harder to steady yourself when the load moves as you shift the bag or walk. Wrap the bag as many times as you can, trim the excess and wrap it all up with duct tape. An old backpack, sack or duffel bag also makes a great outer container for the homemade bag; the garbage bag and duct tape keep the sand inside and you can grip the canvas or burlap material of the various bags much more easily—not to mention you may have some handles to experiment with!

If you'd like to make your bag heavier or lighter, you can fill it with other objects besides sand. Just stay away from really hard fillings like rocks. They're more likely to pinch your fingers, land on your feet or smack you in the head during the movement.

PIGGY BACK

1 Stand up straight with your arms hanging loosely at your sides. Have your partner stand behind you.

2 Bend your knees slightly and have your partner place their arms over your shoulders. Reach straight back with your arms underneath your partner's legs and slowly raise the rider by straightening your legs. Make sure you support their upper body weight.

3 Walk at a fast but stable pace.

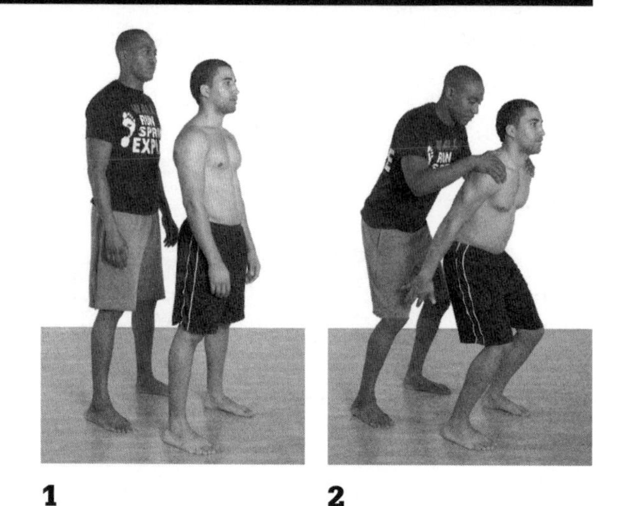

1 **2**

MODIFICATION:
Beginners can use a filled backpack for a lighter load.

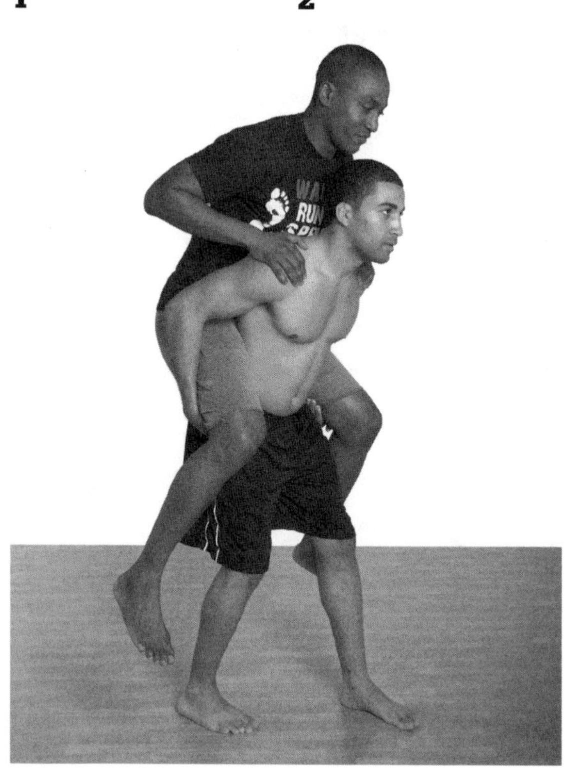

3

FIREMAN'S CARRY

1 Hold your partner's right wrist with your left hand and place it over your right shoulder, across the back.

2 Squat down, keeping a strong and solid back position. Place your right hand behind your partner's right leg and your arm behind their right thigh. Use your leg muscles to rise from the squat and position your partner's right thigh over your right shoulder as you stand up.

3 Keep your back straight and support your partner's body with your shoulders, adjusting the weight to ensure it's evenly distributed across both shoulders.

Cover the distance required. To put your partner down, bend your legs slightly until your partner's feet touch the ground and they are in a safe position.

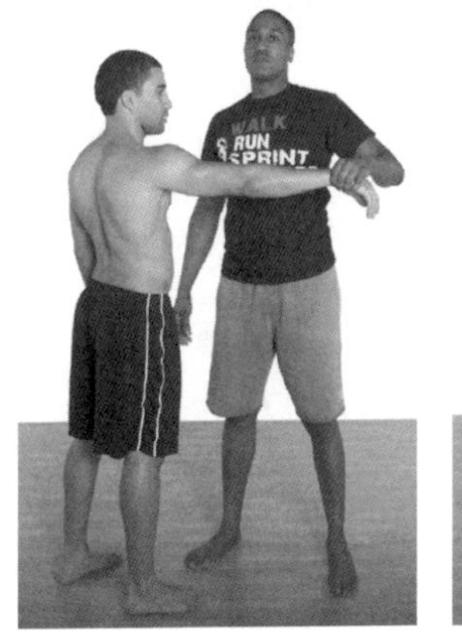

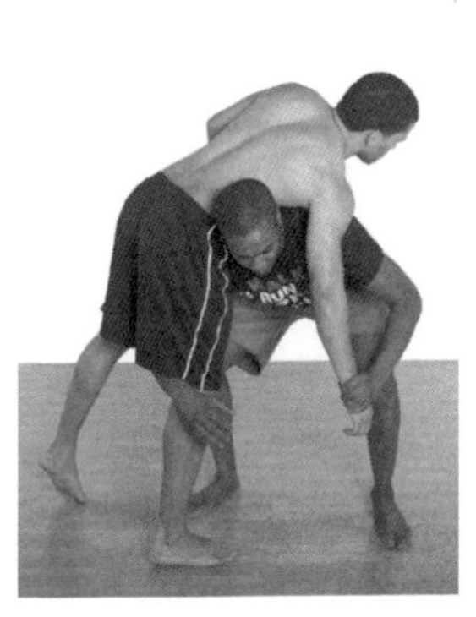

1 **2**

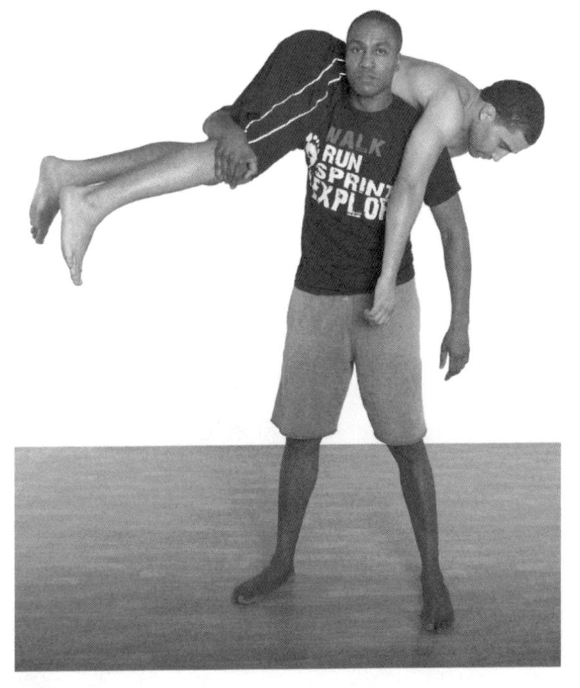

3

FIREMAN'S CARRY SQUAT: Perform a Fireman's Carry and stand up straight with your partner's body weight evenly distributed across your shoulders. Breath in and slowly lower into a low squat position.

Breath in as you rise to a standing position and lift your partner back up.

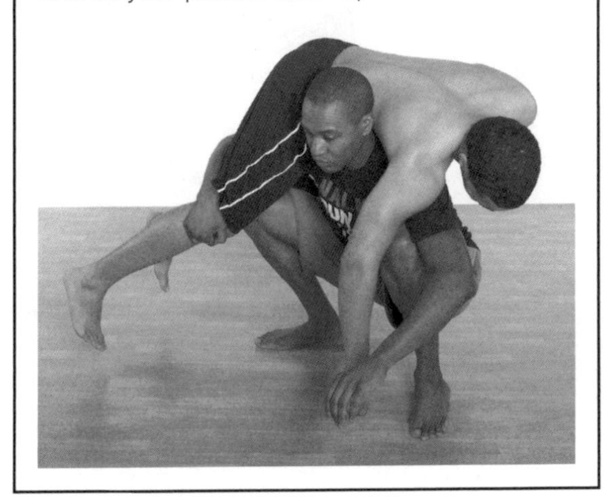

DRACULA CARRY

1 Stand next to our partner with their right arm resting across your shoulders.

2 Place your left arm around your partner's midsection and your right arm under the knee of the leg that's closest to you.

3 Bend your knees slightly, keep your head up, engage your stomach and back muscles, and be sure you can support your partner as they step up or leap up into your arms. Hold and safely carry your partner for the required distance.

To safely lower your partner, bend your knees and keep your back straight. Lower your partner's legs and remove your supporting arms when you are satisfied your partner is stable.

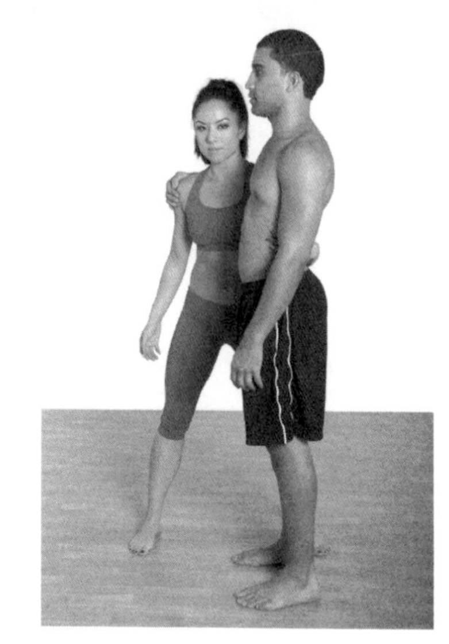

1

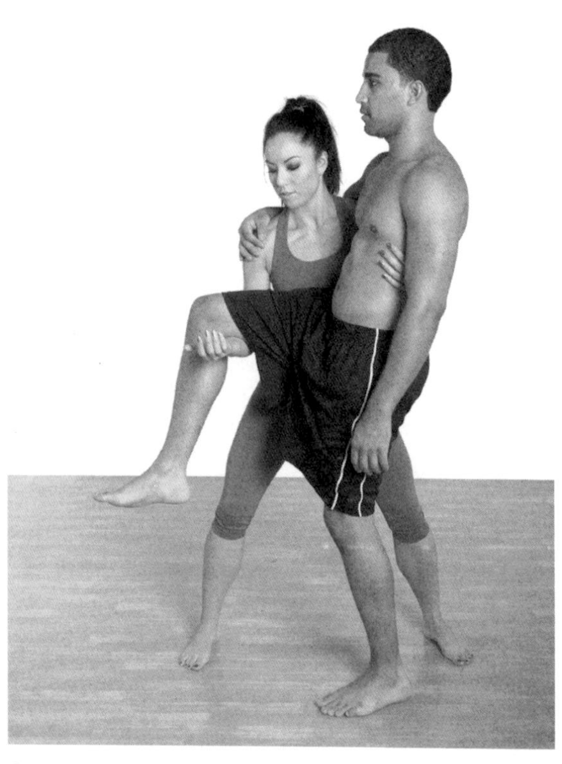

2

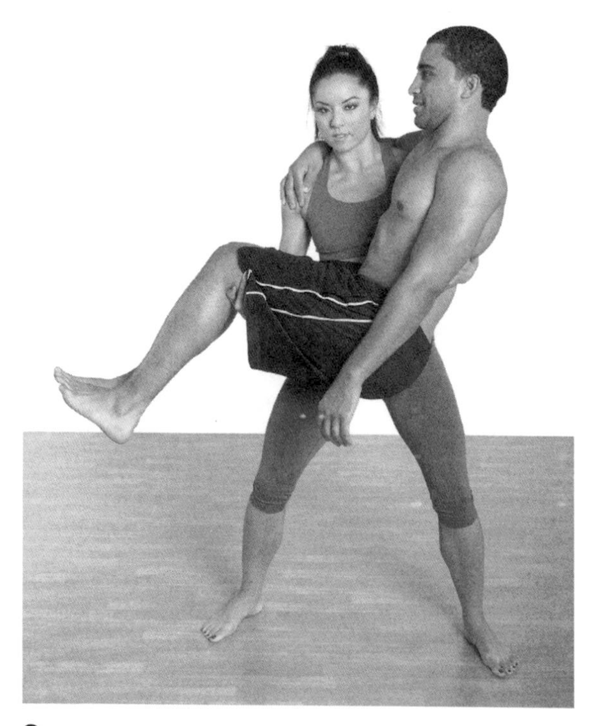

3

DEADLIFT

Many people fear the deadlift, but it has been more appropriately termed the "health lift" in some quarters. A deadlift simply means you're lifting a dead weight, one that isn't moving and is fully supported by the ground before being lifted.

Some people are concerned that deadlifts are not safe for the lower back but, on the contrary, they're probably the best activity for overall back strength. Deadlifts teach you how to keep the lower back strong under a load and are a very practical movement. In fact, what could be more functional? It's just picking something up off the floor in a safe fashion.

You may feel the deadlift is only for weightlifters with a barbell in the gym. However, as always, don't restrict yourself: Use whatever you have at your disposal. You can use a sandbag, log, rock, backpack or whatever is convenient.

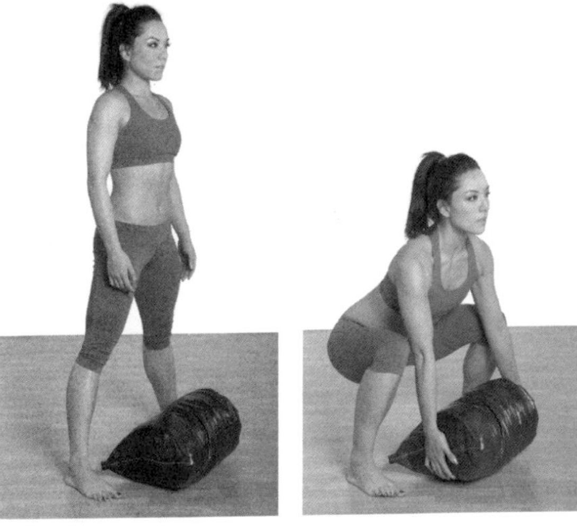

1 **2**

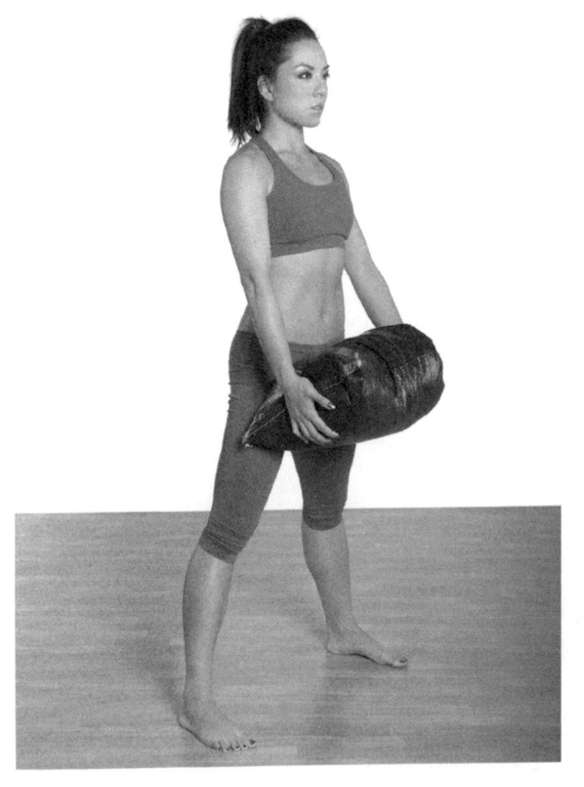

3

1 Stand tall with your feet under your hips and your weight in your heels. Start with your shoulders slightly in front of the object you'll be lifting. Maintain a neutral spine (avoid rounding your back), look straight ahead and brace your core throughout the movement to maintain stability.

2 Keeping your arms extended as long as possible, push your hips back and bend down toward the object.

3 Grasp the object and pick it straight up with your arms fully extended until it's at hip height. Don't pull the object up with your arms.

Return the object to the ground along the same path.

FRONT SQUAT

1 Stand with your feet shoulder-width apart and slightly turned out and hold a sandbag or other weight in your hands.

2 Keep your elbows in tight and the weight close to your body as you descend into the low squat position.

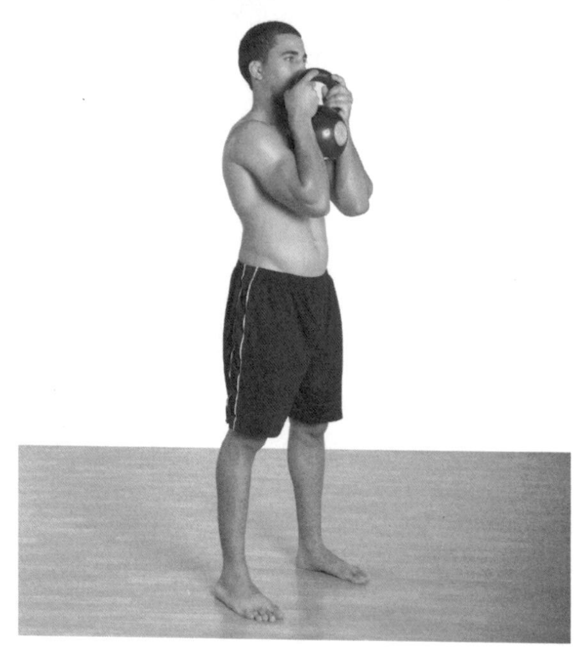

1

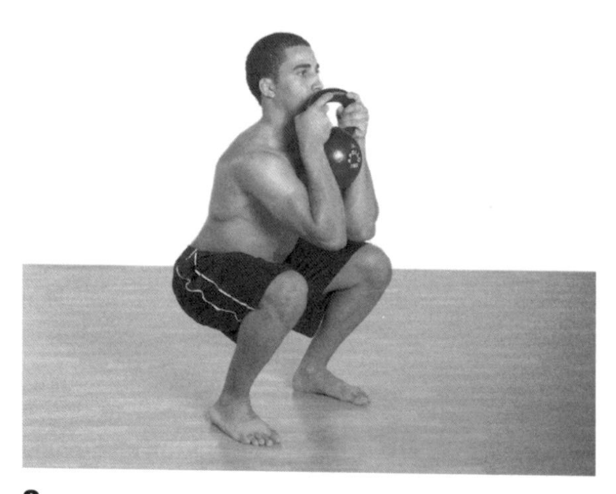

2

PUSH PRESS

1 Stand with your feet shoulder-width apart. Hold a sandbag or other weight in your hands with your palms up.

2 Keeping your torso straight, dip quickly by bending your hips and knees just a few inches.

3 Without pausing at the bottom of the dip, drive up with your legs and hips until your legs are straight. As your legs straighten, press up with your shoulders and arms, passing the sandbag overhead until your arms are fully extended. Maintain a strong midsection throughout and do not overextend your back to get the weight overhead.

Use controlled movement to return the weight to starting position.

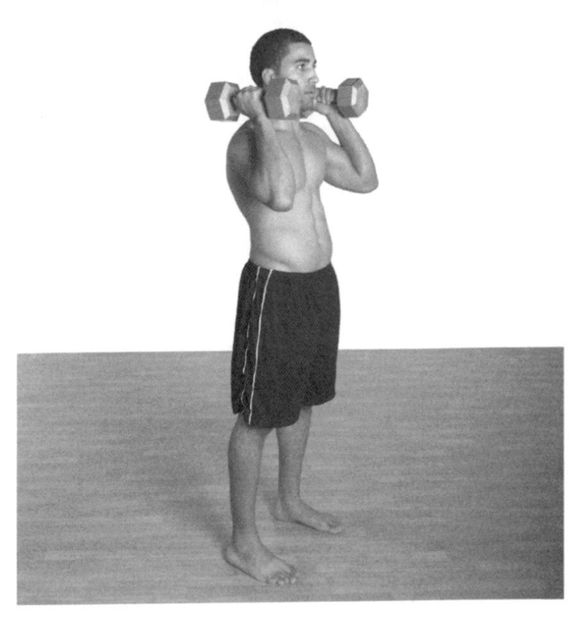

1

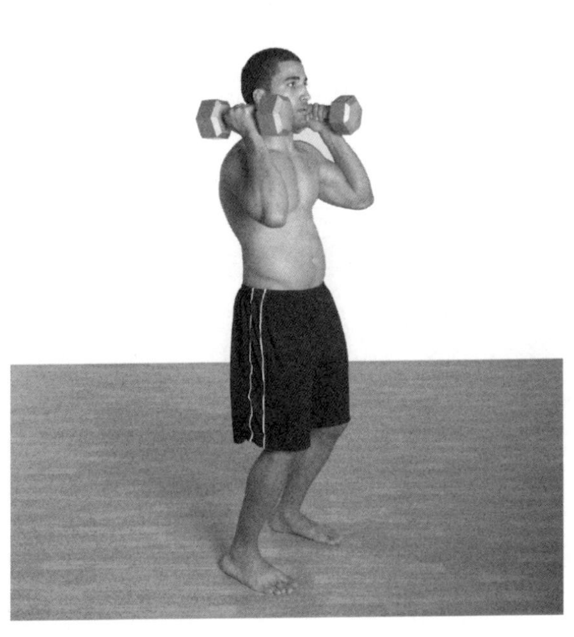

2

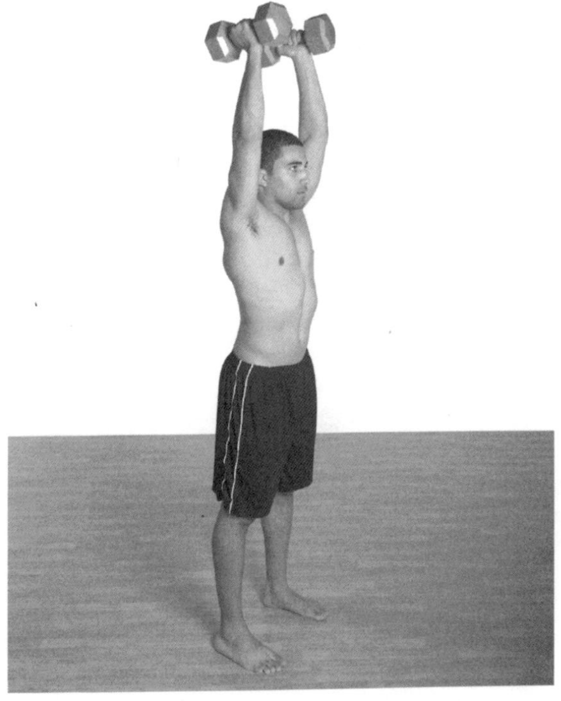

3

SHOULDER-TO-SHOULDER PRESS

1 Stand with your feet shoulder-width apart. Place a sandbag on your right shoulder with both hands on either side of the bag.

2 Press the bag directly up and over your head.

3 Place it down onto your left shoulder.

Return the bag overhead and back to your right shoulder.

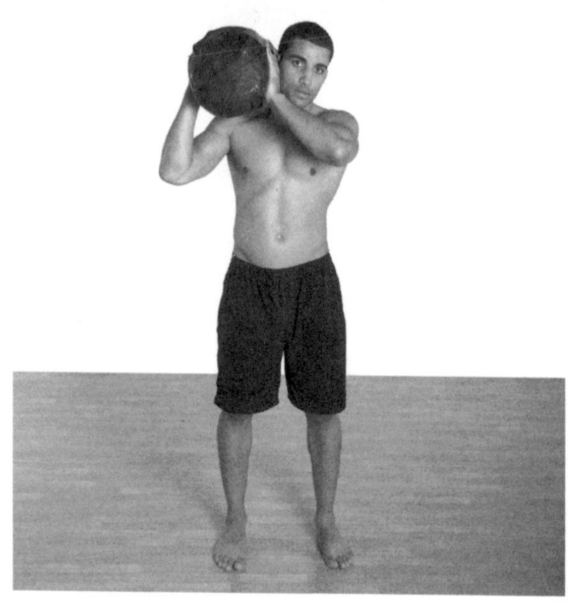

1

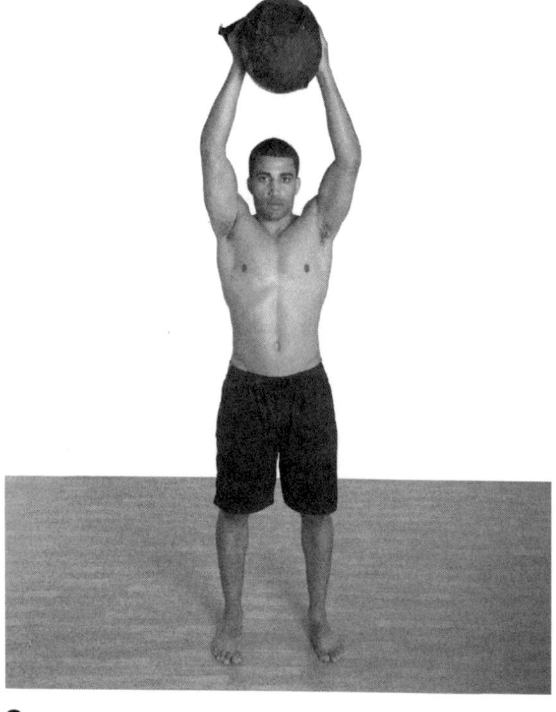

2

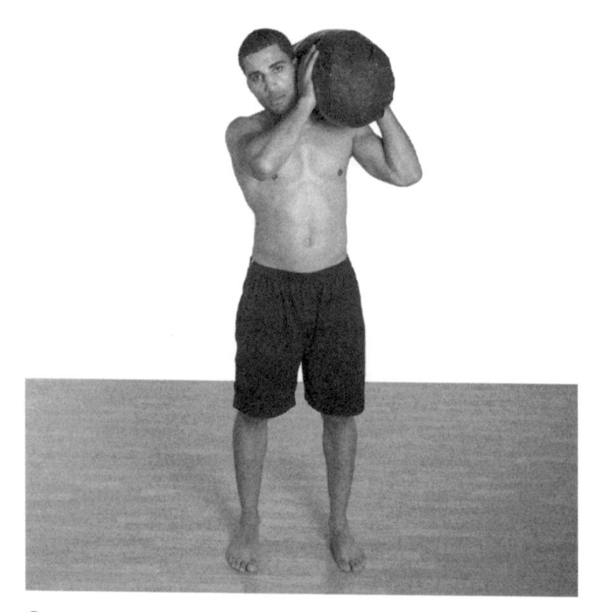

3

FARMER'S WALK

1–2 Pick up two kettlebells, dumbbells, logs or other heavy objects and walk for the specified distance or number of steps.

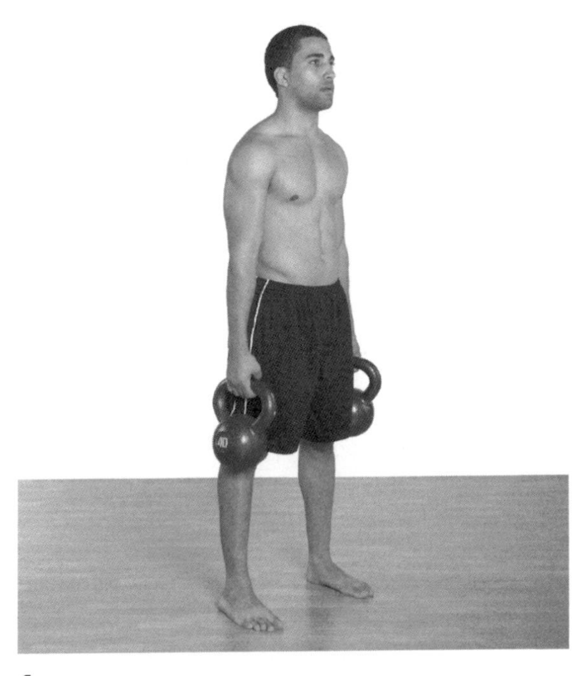

1

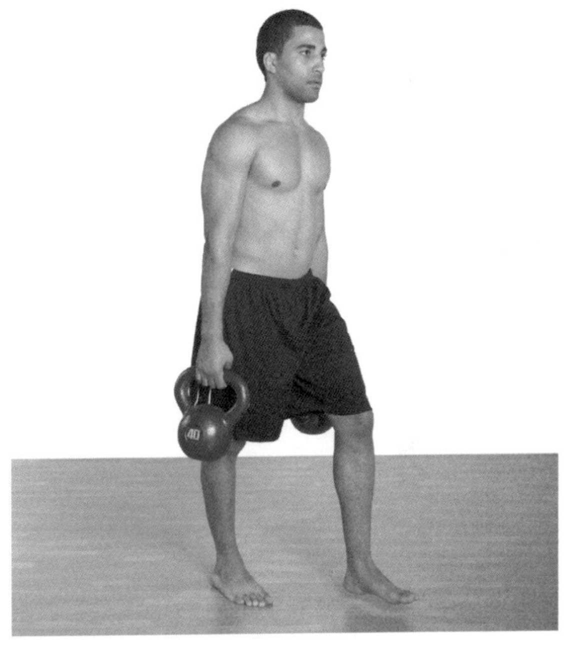

2

WAITER'S WALK

1 Pick up a kettlebell, dumbbell, rock or other heavy object and press it up over your head with one hand.

2 Keeping the arm fully extended and your torso straight and not leaning too far to one side, walk for the specified distance.

Repeat with the other arm.

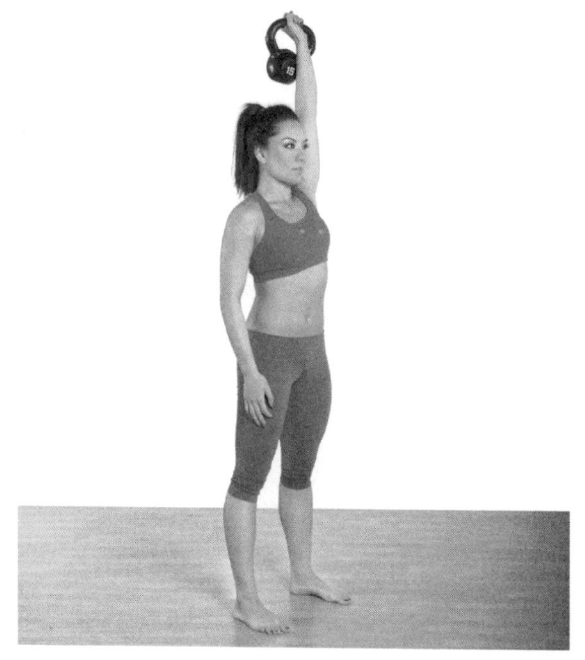

1

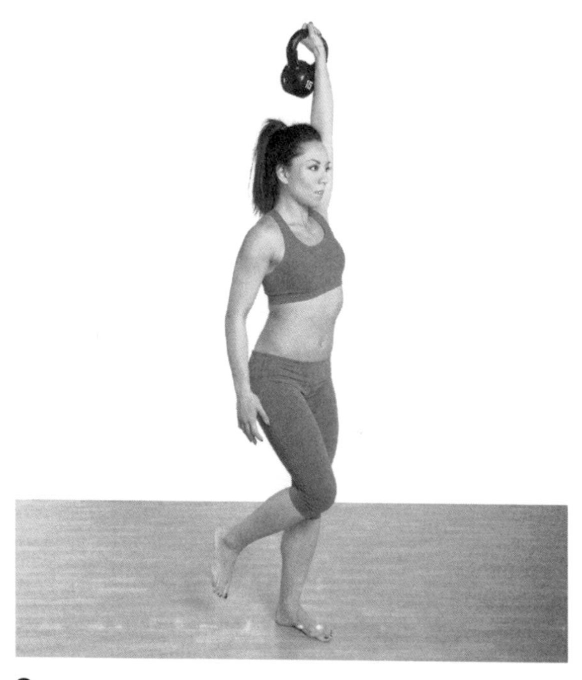

2

OVERHEAD LUNGE

Perform a walking lunge (page 76) but hold an object above your head with both hands. Be sure to use slow and controlled movement. This will really challenge your midsection to keep you and the weight balanced.

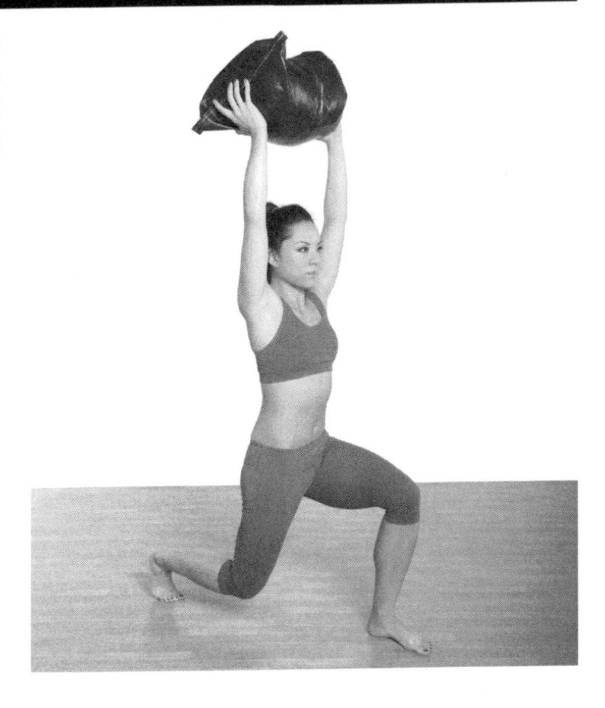

CAR PUSH

This movement is a great way to utilize all the power at your disposal. First make sure someone is steering the car and can apply the brakes. Put the car in neutral and release the parking brake.

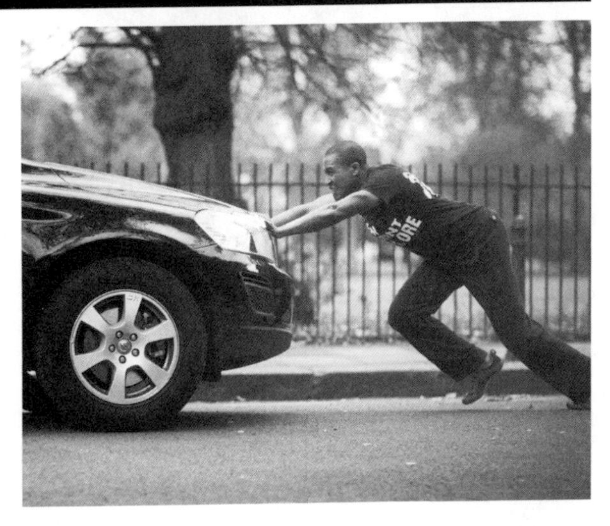

1 Keeping your core tight and your back flat with your hands shoulder-width apart, press your hands against the back of the car. Keep your elbows straight, but don't lock them.

2 Push the car by driving through your lower body from the ground up, making sure you're pushing with your posterior chain (from the backs of your legs, butt and back into your arms) rather than just trying to push with your arms by bending your elbows. Maintain natural breathing throughout.

Cool-Down

The main aim of the cool-down is to promote recovery and return the body to a pre-activity state. Get your heart rate back to normal with controlled breathing by using gentle activity. Any exercise in the Preparation section (page 70) is a good cool-down candidate, as are the specific breathing/relaxation exercises below.

BREATHING/RELAXATION

Breathing is important during movement. We're often only aware when it's pointed out to us that during a period of exertion we're holding our breath. Here are a few exercises that you can use to gain more control over your breathing and aid in bringing relaxation and reducing stress.

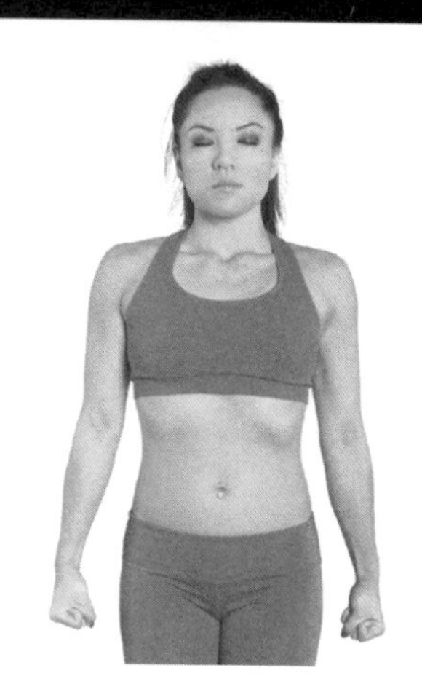

Fist Clench/Diaphragmatic Breathing

Take in a deep breath with your nose and mouth (engage the diaphragm into your breathing rather than just shallowly breathing with your chest). Hold your breath and count to 10 with fists clenched.

Completely and forcefully exhale air from your body as if you were rapidly losing air from a balloon and relax your whole body. This only needs to be performed once.

Full-Body Clench

Create tension by squeezing the muscles in your whole body, from the feet upward, including legs, arms, chest, abs, back, arms, glutes, etc. Hold for a slow count of 10, with controlled breathing.

Slowly release your breath and let your body go completely limp. Repeat 3 to 5 times.

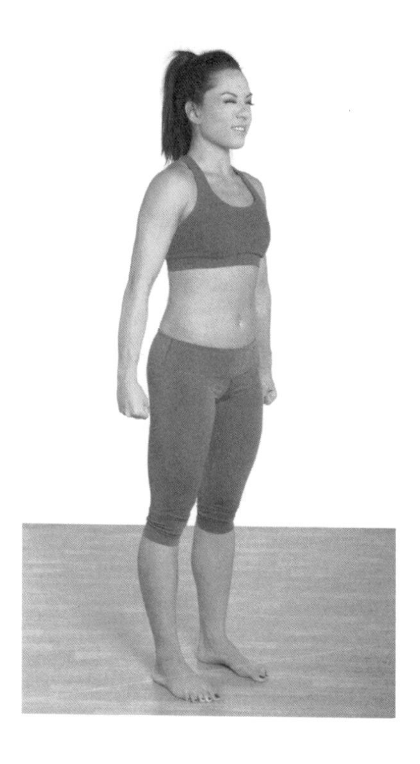

KNEES-APART TOE SQUAT

1 Stand tall with your feet together and your hands clasped behind your head.

2 Push up onto the balls of your feet as high as you can while maintaining balance.

3 Keeping your head up in neutral position and your back straight with a tight midsection, inhale and begin your descent by bending your knees. Open your knees at the bottom of the movement.

Exhale and slowly reverse the movement back up.

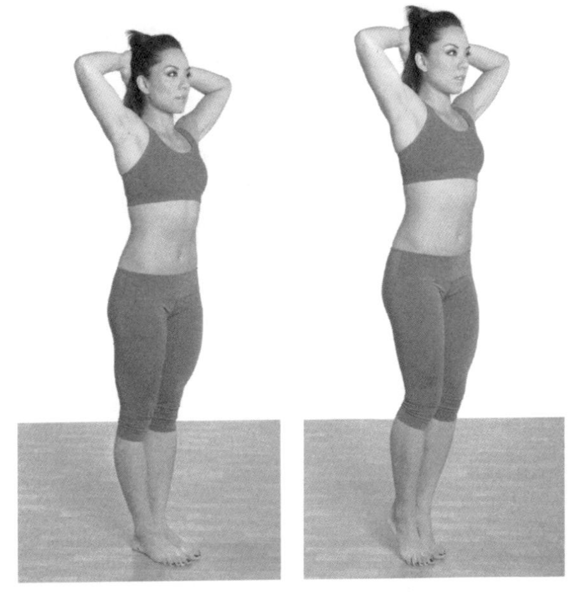

1 **2**

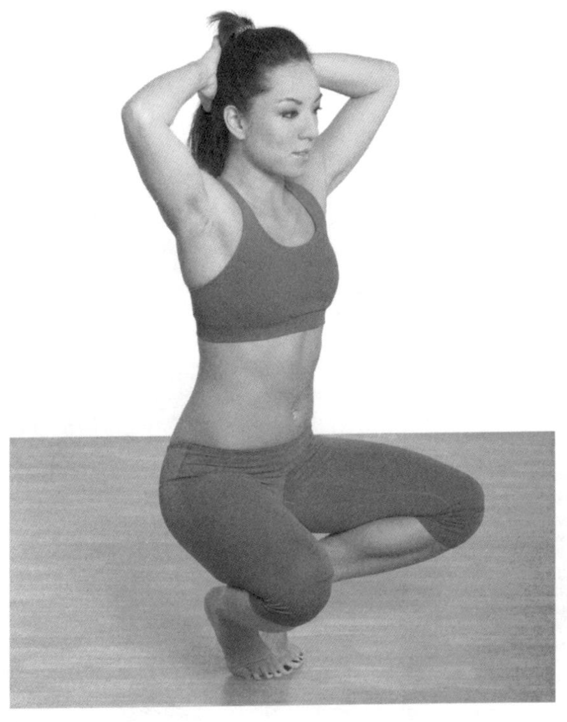

3

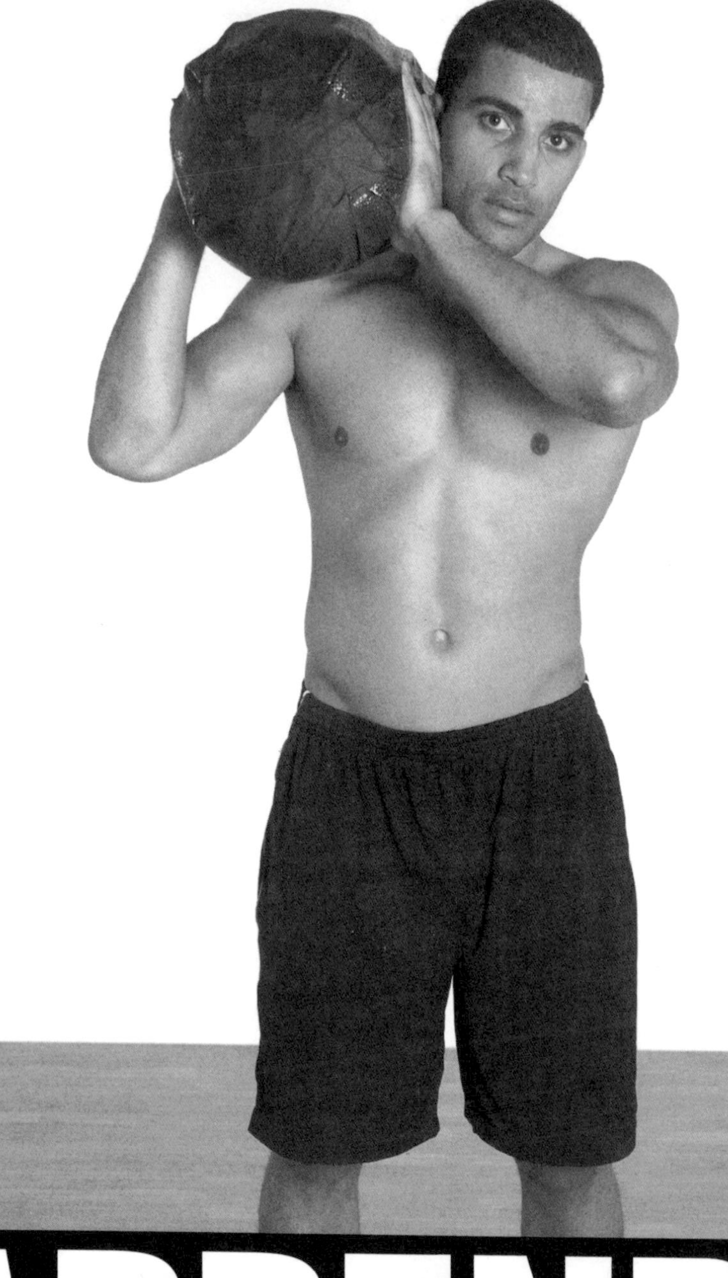

APPENDIX

MEASUREMENTS FOR HEALTH

Body Fat Percentage

A healthy person should be able to burn 1–3 pounds of fat each week while maintaining or increasing lean body tissue. There may be some resistance to begin with as your body adjusts to burning fat as the preferred energy source, but we aim to kick-start this process with the Paleo approach.

As we're focusing on healthy body composition, we need to be aware of your body fat percentage. There are a few methods used to measure the percentage of body fat, some more accurate than others. Three common types of measurement and assessment are BMI, bioelectrical impedance and the use of body fat calipers.

BMI (Body Mass Index)

Often used by the medical profession as an indication of a person's level of fat, this formula is a person's weight in kilos divided by their height in meters squared. For example, if your height is 6'4" (1.92 m) and your weight is 198 pounds (90kg), the calculation would be 90/(1.92 x 1.92) equals a BMI of 24.41.

A BMI of 25 or above is generally classified as overweight, a BMI of 30 or above indicates obesity. There are many reasons why this could be inaccurate as the BMI stats do not differentiate between muscle mass, fat mass or body shape. So, for example, a healthy athlete with a muscular build could be classified as overweight or even obese based on the formula above. Not a reliable indicator of body fat percentage, but a quick and simple method to use.

Body Fat Scales: Bioelectrical Impedance

Body fat scales use the Bioelectrical Impedance Analysis (BIA) technique to estimate body fat percentage as well as muscle mass, hydration levels and bone density. This method measures body composition by sending a low, safe electrical current through the body. The current passes freely through the fluids contained in muscle tissue, but encounters resistance (it's impeded) when it passes through fat tissue.

The resistance of the fat tissue to the current is termed the "bioelectrical impedance." This is then calculated against your height, gender and weight; the scale can then compute you body fat percentage. The readings can change depending on the time of day, activity, hydration levels and whether you have just eaten or not. For consistency it's best to take the reading at the same time of day (mid-afternoon tends to be ideal as a mid-point between lunch and dinner).

Body Fat Calipers

Body fat calipers measure skinfolds at various points of the body to calculate how much subcutaneous fat (fat under the skin) a person has. These numbers are entered into a formula to work out the body fat percentage.

Normally you require an examiner to perform this task, but you can get self-measurement body fat calipers so you can reliably test yourself.

Here's a breakdown of different levels of body fat percentage.

Description	Women (%)	Men (%)
Essential Fat	10–13	2–6
Athletic	14–20	7–13
Average	21–24	14–17
Above Average	25–30	18–25
Overfat	31–34	26–30
Obese	35–39	31–35
Morbidly Obese	> 40	> 36

Waist-to-Hip Ratio

This is the ratio of the circumference of the waist compared to the hip. This ratio is increasingly being used by doctors in preference to BMI as a better measurement of the risk of obesity and cardiovascular disease. This is calculated by dividing the waist measurement by the hip measurement. This is one measure of abdominal fat and it is used as an important indicator for the so-called metabolic syndrome, a common condition that's associated with insulin resistance (diabetes), high blood fats, hypertension and an increased risk for cardiovascular disease. A waist-to-hip ratio of 0.95–0.90 or less is considered healthy for men and a ratio of 0.85–0.80 or less is considered a sign of good health for women. A reading of 1 or higher for both sexes signals an elevated risk and indicates that action should be taken to reduce abdominal fat.

Waist-to-Height Ratio

The waist-to-height ratio is calculated by dividing your waist size by your height. A waist-to-height ratio under <0.5 is generally considered healthy. A value >0.5 indicates an increased risk of developing heart disease and other weight-related conditions. A value >0.6 indicates a significantly increased risk.

Resting Heart Rate (RHR)

Resting heart rate is the number of heart beats per minute your body has while at rest; the normal range is usually between 60 and 80 beats per minute. The resting heart rate can be an indication of your basic fitness level. In most cases, the lower the better. The better trained your body, the less effort and fewer beats per minute it takes your heart to pump blood to your body while at rest. Resting heart rate rises with age or certain medical conditions.

Waist Measurement

If you carry fat mainly around your waist, you're more likely to develop health problems than if you carry fat mainly in your hips and thighs. This is true even if your body fat falls within the normal range. Women with a waist measurement of 35 inches or more and men with a waist measurement of 40 inches or more may have a higher disease risk than people with smaller waist measurements because of where their fat lies.

Blood Pressure

Blood pressure is the pressure of the blood against the walls of the arteries. It's always given as two numbers. The higher (systolic) number represents the pressure while the heart contracts to pump blood to the body. The lower (diastolic) number represents the pressure when the heart relaxes between the beats. Blood pressure of around 110/70 mmHg (millimeters of mercury) is considered optimal for adults. Around 120/80 is considered normal.

"Hypertension" is the term used when your blood pressure remains abnormally high. The primary causes of this condition can be hereditary factors; however, those who are overweight or obese, consume too much salt, eat few fruits and vegetables, drink alcohol and caffeine-rich beverages, smoke, are inactive and have high stress levels all have a higher likelihood of high blood pressure.

Starting Weight & Measurements

DATE: ___________________

Starting Weight: ______________ lbs/kg

RHR: ______________

Blood Pressure: ______________

Body Fat: ______________ %

Starting Waist Measurement: ________ inches/cm

Starting Hip Measurement: ________ inches/cm

Waist-to-Height Ratio: ______________

Waist-to-Hip Ratio: ______________

Notes: ______________

____

Progress

WEEK 1

Weight: ______________ lbs/kg

RHR: ______________

Blood Pressure: ______________

Body Fat (If available): ______________ %

Waist Measurement: ________ inches/cm

Hip Measurement: ________ inches/cm

Waist-to-Height Ratio: ______________

Waist-to-Hip Ratio: ______________

Notes: ______________

____

WEEK 2

Weight: ______________ lbs/kg

RHR: ______________

Blood Pressure: ______________

Body Fat (If available): ______________ %

Waist Measurement: ________ inches/cm

Hip Measurement: ________ inches/cm

Waist-to-Height Ratio: ______________

Waist-to-Hip Ratio: ______________

Notes: ______________

____

WEEK 3

Weight: ______________ lbs/kg

RHR: ______________

Blood Pressure: ______________

Body Fat (If available): ______________ %

Waist Measurement: ________ inches/cm

Hip Measurement: ________ inches/cm

Waist-to-Height Ratio: ______________

Waist-to-Hip Ratio: ______________

Notes: ______________

____

WEEK 4

Weight: ______________ lbs/kg

RHR: ______________

Blood Pressure: ______________

Body Fat (If available): ______________ %

Waist Measurement: ________ inches/cm

Hip Measurement: ________ inches/cm

Waist-to-Height Ratio: ______________

Waist-to-Hip Ratio: ______________

Notes: ______________

____

WEEK 5

Weight: ______________________lbs/kg

RHR: ______________________

Blood Pressure: ______________________

Body Fat (If available): ______________ %

Waist Measurement: ____________ inches/cm

Hip Measurement: ____________ inches/cm

Waist-to-Height Ratio: ______________________

Waist-to-Hip Ratio: ______________________

Notes: ______________________

____

WEEK 6

Weight: ______________________lbs/kg

RHR: ______________________

Blood Pressure: ______________________

Body Fat (If available): ______________ %

Waist Measurement: ____________ inches/cm

Hip Measurement: ____________ inches/cm

Waist-to-Height Ratio: ______________________

Waist-to-Hip Ratio: ______________________

Notes: ______________________

____

WEEK 7

Weight: ______________________lbs/kg

RHR: ______________________

Blood Pressure: ______________________

Body Fat (If available): ______________ %

Waist Measurement: ____________ inches/cm

Hip Measurement: ____________ inches/cm

Waist-to-Height Ratio: ______________________

Waist-to-Hip Ratio: ______________________

Notes: ______________________

____

WEEK 8

Weight: ______________________lbs/kg

RHR: ______________________

Blood Pressure: ______________________

Body Fat (If available): ______________ %

Waist Measurement: ____________ inches/cm

Hip Measurement: ____________ inches/cm

Waist-to-Height Ratio: ______________________

Waist-to-Hip Ratio: ______________________

Notes: ______________________

____

RECIPES

CARIBBEAN FISH STEW

This dish would be delicious with a side of Swoon-Worthy Sweet Potatoes (page 145).

- 2 Tbsp. extra-virgin coconut oil, divided
- 1 lb. cod fillets, skinned and cut into bite-size pieces (or use other firm, non-flaky white fish like monkfish, mahi mahi, haddock, halibut, etc.)
- ½ c. finely minced shallot (about 2 large shallots)
- 2 Tbsp. finely minced garlic (about 4 large cloves)
- 2 Tbsp. fresh ginger, peeled and finely minced (about a 2-in. piece)
- ½ c. diced celery
- 1 large fresh bay leaf
- 6 c. water, divided
- 1 (13.5-oz.) can coconut milk
- 3 c. diced vine-ripened tomatoes (about 7 large tomatoes)
- 1 Tbsp. seeded, diced Scotch Bonnet pepper (about 1 small pepper)
- 1 c. red bell pepper (about ¾ large pepper)
- 1 c. green bell pepper (about ¾ large pepper)
- 1 c. sliced okra, sliced crosswise into ¼-in. rounds
- ¼ tsp. ground allspice
- 1 tsp. saffron threads
- ¼ tsp. ground black pepper, or to taste
- ½ Tbsp. fresh thyme leaves
- 2 Tbsp. freshly squeezed lime juice
- ¼ c. fresh cilantro, finely minced

In a large (12–13-in.) sauté pan, heat 1 Tbsp. of the extra-virgin coconut oil over high heat until shimmering. Reduce the heat to medium high, then add the cod fillet pieces and sauté 5 minutes per side, or until crisp and golden brown. Meanwhile, in a large (6–8-qt.) stock pot, heat the remaining extra-virgin coconut oil over high heat until shimmering. Reduce the heat to low, then add the shallots, garlic, ginger, celery and bay leaf, and sauté for 5 minutes, or until tender, stirring occasionally. Deglaze with ¼ cup of the water, scrape off the fond (the brown bits on the bottom of the pan), then add the remaining 5¾ c. water and the coconut milk and bring to a rolling boil, covering with a lid so it boils faster. Remove the lid, reduce to medium-low heat then stir in the tomatoes and simmer, uncovered, for 10 minutes. Add the sautéed cod fillet pieces, Scotch Bonnet pepper, red and green bell peppers, okra, ground allspice, saffron, ground black pepper and thyme leaves. Then cover again and simmer for 5–7 more minutes, or until vegetables are tender but still retain their color. Remove from the heat, uncover and allow to cool for 10 minutes. Discard the bay leaf, add the lime juice, stir and adjust the seasonings to your liking. Garnish with fresh cilantro, and serve immediately.

Yield: About 3 qts. (12 c.), or 6 servings (of 2 c. per person)

SPICY CHICKEN WINGS

2 lbs. chicken wings (about 12 wings), rinsed and drained

6 Tbsp. walnut oil

¼ c. freshly squeezed lemon juice

1 Tbsp. garlic powder

2 Tbsp. ground cumin

2 Tbsp. paprika

4 tsp. dried oregano

2 tsp. ground ginger

½ tsp. ground black pepper

½ tsp. cayenne pepper

Place the prepped chicken wings on a large plate and pat dry with paper towels. Diagonally slash the wings with a sharp knife. Transfer to a large zip-top bag, add all remaining ingredients, seal and gently shake the bag to combine. Massage the chicken from outside the bag to evenly distribute spices and rub them into chicken, including the slashes and crevices. Refrigerate overnight.

To cook on the grill: Preheat a grill to medium-high heat. Place the wings on the grill, close the grill lid and cook about 20 minutes total or until juices run clear when pierced with a fork, turning them over once after the first 10 minutes. Serve immediately. To cook in the oven: Preheat the oven to 350°F. Bake wings for 20 minutes total or until juices run clear when pierced with a fork, turning them over once after the first 10 minutes. Serve immediately.

Yield: 12 wings, 3–4 servings

SWOON-WORTHY SWEET POTATOES

1 lb. scrubbed, diced, unpeeled sweet potatoes (about 2 medium potatoes; makes about 3 c. diced)

3 Tbsp. walnut oil

2 Tbsp. freshly squeezed lemon juice

1 Tbsp. paprika

1 tsp. cracked black pepper, or to taste

2 Tbsp. fresh Tuscan Blue rosemary, finely minced (about 2 small sprigs)

1½ Tbsp. finely minced garlic (about 3 large cloves)

½ c. finely minced shallots (about 2 large shallots)

2 Tbsp. fresh oregano, finely minced (about 1 small sprig)

2 Tbsp. fresh thyme (about 2 large sprigs)

2 Tbsp. finely minced fresh Italian flat-leaf parsley

Place all the ingredients, except for the oregano, thyme and parsley, into a large bowl in the exact order given, and toss with a spatula or large serving spoon until the potatoes are fully coated. Next, heat a large (12–13-in.) sauté pan for about 30 seconds over medium-high heat, then reduce the heat to medium and add the sweet potato mixture, evenly distributing the potatoes across the pan. Cook for 10 minutes, then add the oregano and thyme and cook for another 10 minutes, stirring frequently. Add the parsley and cook for 2–3 minutes longer, or until the potatoes are tender and golden brown. Remove from the heat, garnish with a few sprigs of fresh parsley and serve immediately.

Yield: 4 servings

CAULIFLOWER MASH

This dish is a great comfort food, and it's incredibly nutritious to boot. Cauliflower mash goes amazingly well with all sorts of main courses, particularly chicken, turkey, fish, beef and lamb.

- 1 medium unpeeled garlic clove (makes about ¾ tsp. mashed, roasted garlic)
- 1 Tbsp. walnut oil, plus more for roasting garlic
- 1 head cauliflower (about 1 lb.), quartered and then broken into florets
- 1 tsp. dried rosemary
- ¼ tsp. paprika
- ⅛ tsp. ground black pepper
- ⅛ tsp. ground nutmeg

Preheat a toaster oven to 400°F. Place the unpeeled garlic clove on a small piece of aluminum foil, then drizzle with a small amount of walnut oil. Completely wrap the garlic in the foil, then place on the toaster oven tray and roast for 25–30 minutes, or until golden brown. Meanwhile, place a steamer basket in a large pot, fill the pot with water until it reaches the bottom of the basket and then bring to a rolling boil. Add the cauliflower florets, cover and boil for 15–20 minutes, or until the cauliflower is tender. Drain the cauliflower into a colander and let it rest there for 1–2 minutes to dry. When the garlic has finished roasting, remove it from toaster oven and let cool for 5 minutes, or until cool to the touch. Then peel and mash. Measure out ¾ tsp. of the mashed garlic and place this amount into a food processor, followed by the steamed cauliflower. Add the remaining ingredients, and process until fluffy. Serve immediately.

Yield: 4–6 servings

SHIRAZI SALAD

This Persian salad from where else but the region of Shiraz is quite simple and quick to make. It's sort of like a Persian pico de gallo. This no-cook dish consists of only three vegetables: tomatoes, cucumbers and onions. Typically served in the summer, this salad goes particularly well with other side dishes like baba ganoush or grilled shish-kebabs, like chicken.

½ c. diced red onion (about ½ small red onion)

1½ c. Persian or English (seedless) cucumber, unpeeled, scored lengthwise with a fork, diced and then measured (about 1½ Persian cucumbers or 1 medium English cucumber)

1½ c. diced and drained vine-ripened tomatoes (about 2 medium tomatoes)

2 Tbsp. finely chopped fresh mint (or 1 tsp. dried mint, if fresh is unavailable)

¼ c. freshly squeezed lime juice (from about 2 large limes)

2 Tbsp walnut oil

⅛ tsp. ground black pepper, or to taste

2 tsp. ground sumac (be sure to use salt-free variety)

Combine the onion, cucumbers, tomatoes and mint in a large bowl and set aside. Combine the lime juice, walnut oil, black pepper and sumac in a blender and pulse until well-combined. Pour the dressing on top of the salad and toss until the vegetables are completely coated with dressing. Cover and refrigerate for at least 30 minutes before serving. Serve cold.

Chef's Note: Be sure to dice the onion first, followed by the cucumbers, and finally the tomatoes, in that particular order, to keep your cutting board as dry as possible. Also, try to dice the vegetables to a uniform size.

To make this dish into a main course, simply add a protein like grilled chicken, lamb or beef.

Sumac can be purchased at most Middle Eastern or Mediterranean markets. If you don't have a local resource, you can always purchase it online.

Yield: 4 servings

SPAGHETTI SQUASH & SPICY MEATBALLS

3 lbs. spaghetti squash, halved crosswise (about 1 medium squash)

Meatballs:

½ lb. lean ground turkey

½ lb. lean ground beef

¼ c. finely minced fresh spinach

2 eggs

¼ tsp. ground black pepper, or to taste

½ tsp. dried basil

2 Tbsp. finely minced fresh Italian flat-leaf parsley

½ tsp. dried oregano

½ tsp. garlic powder

½ tsp. onion powder

2 tsp. paprika

¼ tsp. ground cayenne pepper

Tomato Sauce (makes 32 oz.):

1 c. diced yellow onion (about ½ onion)

2 Tbsp. peeled and finely minced garlic (about 4 large cloves)

4 c. diced vine-ripened tomatoes (about 3 large tomatoes)

1 c. water, or more as needed

¼ tsp. ground black pepper

¼ c. minced fresh basil, densely packed, plus more for garnish

1 Tbsp. finely minced fresh oregano, densely packed

1 Tbsp. finely minced fresh marjoram, densely packed

2 Tbsp. finely minced fresh Italian flat-leaf parsley, densely packed

Preheat the oven to 375°F. Next, bring a large pot of water to a rolling boil, and then carefully place the halved squash into the pot, using a sturdy pair of tongs, and boil for 20 to 25 minutes, or until tender. Let the squash cool for at least 10 minutes before handling. Then, using a large spoon, scoop out the pulp and seeds and discard. Separate the spaghetti squash strands with a fork, scraping with the grain of the noodles (crosswise). Use the same spoon you just used to scrape out all of the strands to remove the spaghetti squash strands en masse. Once you've loosened some of the strands, it'll be easier to insert your spoon closer to the rind and excavate the remainder. If you've cooked the squash for long enough, this should be relatively easy to do. Divide up the squash into four portions and place into bowls.

Meanwhile, place all of the meatball ingredients in a large bowl and thoroughly mix together using a spatula or fork. Using a cookie dough scoop (or small ice cream scoop), form bite-size meatballs and place as many as will fit into a large ovenproof skillet, cooking them in multiple batches until all meatballs have been cooked. (No extra oil is needed, as the rendered fat from the meat will provide adequate liquid fat to brown the meatballs and keep them from burning. If needed, you can always add a bit of water during cooking.) Place the meatballs into the oven and bake for 15 minutes total, or until golden brown. Then transfer the skillet from the oven to the stovetop, and sear the meatballs over high heat for an additional 5 minutes, browning them on all sides. Remove from the heat, drain the fat from the pan and let cool for several minutes. Using a slotted spoon, divide the meatballs into equal portions and place on top of each bowl of squash. Set aside.

Next, make the tomato sauce: In a medium pot over high heat, combine the onions, garlic, tomatoes and water and bring to a boil, then reduce the heat and simmer for 10 minutes, stirring frequently. (If the mixture cooks down too quickly, reduce heat a bit and/or add more water as needed.) Season with pepper, and then stir to fully incorporate. Add all of the fresh herbs (basil, oregano, marjoram and parsley) and continue to cook for another 5 minutes. Remove from the heat and then pour the sauce over meatballs and squash. Garnish with additional basil, if desired. Serve hot.

Yield: 4 servings

JAMAICAN JERK CHICKEN WITH GRILLED GREEN PLANTAINS

5 lbs. whole bone-in chicken, cut into pieces (wings, breasts, drumsticks, etc.) and trimmed of fat

¼ c. sliced scallions, cut crosswise into ¼-in.-thick rounds (for garnish)

Jerk Sauce:

1 c. coarsely chopped scallions

½ c. diced red onion

2 Tbsp. minced garlic (about 4 large cloves)

3 Scotch Bonnet peppers halved, stemmed and seeded (if unavailable, substitute 3 habañero chile peppers or, for mild chicken, half a red bell pepper)

¼ c. freshly squeezed lime juice

3 Tbsp. extra-virgin coconut oil

2 Tbsp. fresh peeled and diced ginger (about a 2-in. piece)

2 Tbsp. fresh thyme leaves

1 Tbsp. ground allspice

1 Tbsp. ground cinnamon

1 Tbsp. ground coriander

1 tsp. ground cloves

1 tsp. ground nutmeg

½ tsp. ground black pepper

Seasoned Smoke:

3 Ceylon cinnamon sticks (about 3 in. each)

50 whole allspice berries

1 handful pimento (a.k.a. allspice) wood chips or sticks (optional; if unavailable, use pecan, pear or oak wood chips)

1 c. (or more) water (for soaking seasoned smoke ingredients)

Grilled Plantains:

2 Tbsp. extra-virgin coconut oil

2 c. thinly sliced green plantains (about 2 large plantains)

2 Tbsp. unsweetened shredded coconut

⅛ tsp. ground black pepper, or to taste

Place the chicken on a large, nonporous cutting board. Poke holes all over the chicken with a sharp knife, place it in a large zip-top plastic bag and set aside. Combine all of the jerk sauce ingredients in a food processor and pulse until smooth. Pour the jerk sauce into the zip-top bag containing the chicken, reserving about ½ c. to use for basting. Seal the bag and thoroughly massage the spice mix into the chicken from the outside of the bag. Marinate overnight in the refrigerator. Thirty minutes before grilling, remove the chicken from the refrigerator and let rest until it reaches room temperature. Preheat a grill to medium-high heat. For the seasoned smoke, soak the cinnamon sticks, allspice berries and wood chips in a bowl of water for 10 minutes. Make an aluminum foil "boat," curling up foil ends and fastening them together to secure. Remove the sticks, berries, and chips from the bowl of water, drain and place them in the aluminum foil "boat." Place chicken and foil boat on the grill, close the grill lid and grill the chicken for about 15 minutes per side, or until the juices run clear when pierced with a fork. After the first 15 minutes, baste the chicken with the reserved sauce before you flip it over. Transfer to a large serving platter and let rest 10–15 minutes before slicing.

While the chicken is resting, make the plantains: Heat the coconut oil over high heat in a large (12–13-in.) sauté pan until glistening. Reduce the heat to medium-low, then add sliced the plantains and cook for about 3–5 minutes per side, or until golden brown. In the last 2 minutes of cooking, sprinkle the shredded coconut on top of the plantains and stir to combine. Remove from the heat and divide among 4 plates. To serve, place the chicken on the plates alongside the plantains. Garnish the chicken with ¼ c. sliced scallions. Serve and enjoy!

Yield: 6–8 servings

PAN-GRILLED BABY LAMB CHOPS WITH FRESH HERBS

1 lb. lamb chops, Frenched, then washed, patted dry and trimmed of fat

1½ Tbsp. fresh rosemary, very finely minced

1 Tbsp. fresh thyme, very finely minced

½ Tbsp. fresh oregano, very finely minced

2 Tbsp. fresh minced Italian flat leaf parsley

1–2 tsp. freshly squeezed lemon juice, or to taste

1 tsp. freshly cracked black pepper

¼ c. very finely minced shallots (about 1 large shallot)

1 Tbsp. very finely minced garlic (about 2 large cloves)

½ c. water, divided, or more as needed

When you're prepping the lamb, be sure to leave a thin layer of surface fat remaining on the top face (i.e., meat side of the chops; this helps preserve the meat's tenderness) and diagonally score the fatty side of each chop by making shallow cuts through the remaining surface fat, spacing each cut about a ½ in. apart.

Combine the rosemary, thyme, oregano and parsley in a small bowl and set aside. Place the lamb chops in a large zip-top plastic bag, pour the lemon juice over top and season all over with black pepper followed by the herb mixture you just made. Seal the bag and marinate overnight. One hour before you plan to cook the lamb, remove the lamb chops from the refrigerator and allow them to reach room temperature. (This ensures even heat distribution during cooking.)

Place a large (12 to 13-in.) sauté pan over medium heat for 60 seconds. Place the chops into the pan and sear on all four sides for 3 to 4 minutes per side (for medium rare), or until golden brown. (Cook 2 to 2½ minutes per side for rare.) To sear the bottom side of the chops, hold each set of chops upright (i.e., vertically) and then tilt them in various configurations in order to cook them on the remaining sides. If you don't want to cook them in batches, which takes a lot longer, lean them upright against the interior sides of the pan (for hands-free support), so you can cook the bottom sides of the chops and still have a free hand to scrape off the fond (i.e., the "brown bits" that form on the bottom of the pan) to keep it from burning.

Right before searing the fourth and final side of the lamb chops, add the shallots and garlic to the pan and sauté them alongside the chops. (No added oil is needed as the rendered fat from the chops will provide more than adequate liquid fat to cook the vegetables.) As soon as the garlic and shallots begin to brown, deglaze the pan by adding ¼ c. water at a time, waiting until each portion of liquid cooks down before adding the next. (Add as much water as necessary to keep the liquid in the pan from drying up and the fond from burning. The pan should never become dry during cooking.)

Remove the pan from the heat and allow chops to cool until they can be safely handled. Let the lamb rest for 5–10 minutes before slicing into a chop to check for doneness. The temperature of the meat will climb an additional 10 degrees as it rests, which is just perfect for the final resting temperature for medium rare.) To serve, transfer four chops to each plate and drizzle with jus from the pan and some lemon juice, if desired. For visual impact, surround the lamb with steamed or sautéed vegetables in a decorative fashion.

Yield: 2 servings

MUSHROOM PEPPER STEAK

Steak:

1 tsp. freshly cracked black pepper

2 tsp. fennel seeds

2 tsp. garlic powder

1 (8-oz.) steak filet (about ¾ to 1 in. thick), at room temperature (remove from the refrigerator at least 30 minutes before grilling)

Sautéed Mushrooms:

1 Tbsp. avocado oil

¼ c. peeled and finely minced shallots (about 1 large shallot)

1 c. quartered mushrooms

pinch of ground black pepper, or to taste

⅛ c. water (or beef stock)

1 tsp. fresh thyme

Preheat a grill to high. Mix together all steak ingredients except the steak (cracked black pepper, fennel seeds, and garlic) in a small bowl. Put the steak on a large plate, then sprinkle the spice mix on top. Use tongs to flip the steak over, then season on the other side. Then place the fillet onto its side and gently press it into the remaining spices on the plate, rotating it around until all sides have been thoroughly spiced, and place onto the hot grill. Grill the steak with the grill lid closed, for 3–4 minutes per side for medium rare, 2–2½ minutes for rare, or until desired temperature has been reached. (Remember that once it's done, the steak's temperature will continue to rise a few more degrees as it rests, so be sure not to overcook your steak.) At about the halfway point, cut into the steak with a fork and knife to check for doneness, and flip to the other side when ready. When done, remove from the heat and let rest on a heatproof plate for 5 minutes before serving. Divide the steak into 2 portions and place onto dinner plates.

While the steak is resting, heat the avocado oil in a large (12–13-in.) sauté pan and warm over medium heat for about 60 seconds. Then reduce the heat to low, add the shallots and sauté for about 2 minutes, or until translucent. Add the mushrooms, sprinkle with pepper (from 10–12 in. or so above, for even distribution) and sauté until tender, about 5 more minutes. Then deglaze with water (or beef stock), stirring continually, and cook for another 5–6 minutes, or until the mushrooms are golden brown. In the last 3 minutes of cooking time, add the fresh thyme leaves and stir to combine. Remove from the heat and serve while hot, alongside or on top of the steak. Enjoy!

Yield: 1 to 2 servings

T'IBS WE'T (ETHIOPIAN BEEF STIR-FRY)

T'ibs w'et is a traditional Ethiopian dish made with beef, red onions and berbere spices, a mixture typically including ginger, clove, coriander, allspice and chile peppers. The exact ingredients and specific quantities used in berbere can vary quite widely, depending on originating region and individual chefs' preferences.

1 lb. flank steak, cut into 1-in. cubes

3¾ tsp. plus a pinch Berbere Spice Mix (recipe follows), divided

1 Tbsp. avocado oil

1 c. red onion, sliced into ¼-in.-thick crescent slivers (about ¾ medium onion)

2 Tbsp. peeled and finely minced garlic (about 4 large cloves)

¼ c. water

1 c. diced vine-ripened tomato (about 1½ large tomatoes)

1 Tbsp. diced seeded jalapeño pepper (about ¼ large pepper)

Berbere Spice Mix:
(Yield: 3¾ tsp. plus a pinch)

½ tsp. ground ginger

½ tsp. ground cardamom

¼ tsp. ground coriander

½ tsp. ground fenugreek

⅛ tsp. ground nutmeg

dash of ground cloves

dash of ground cinnamon

dash of ground allspice

¼ tsp. ground cayenne pepper

¼ tsp. ground black pepper

¼ tsp. ajwain seeds (can be found at an ethnic grocery store or bought online)

1 tsp. paprika

Place the beef and all of the berbere spice mix into a large zip-top plastic bag, seal and marinate overnight. Thirty minutes before cooking, remove the meat and allow to rest until it reaches room temperature. Place a wok or other large pan over high heat. (Since this is a stir-fry, you'll need to use a pan that can withstand and retain high heat.) Add the avocado oil to the pan, followed by the onions and garlic and stir quickly, making sure that ingredients don't brown or burn. Cook the onions and garlic until tender, about 5 minutes. Add the water to the pan, stirring to remove the fond (brown bits) from the bottom. Continue to cook until the water has been reduced by half. Next, add the beef. If you don't hear a sizzle when the steak hits the pan, the pan isn't hot enough. The meat will cook fairly quickly. Be sure to allow enough room in the pan to cook all the ingredients evenly. Next add the diced tomatoes and jalapeño and keep stirring. Cook the steak 3–4 minutes per side, or until the desired level of doneness has been reached. Remove from the heat, let rest a few minutes and serve.

Yield: 3 to 4 servings

MONKFISH IN VERACRUZ SAUCE

From a nutritional standpoint, there are several reasons to eat monkfish. First of all, this fish is high in protein and low in fat, but most of that fat is monounsaturated and polyunsaturated fat, and includes a high amount of omega-3s, the heart-healthy fatty acids that reduce inflammation. In fact, a 3-oz. serving of monkfish provides over 100 mg of omega-3s, more than hamburger, steak, chicken, turkey or pork. One serving contains around 19 g protein, 3 g fat and less than 1 g carbohydrate. This lean, high-protein fish is great for helping the body build and repair muscle as well as produce antibodies, enzymes and hormones. And serving it with Veracruz sauce, a spicy Mexican sauce, makes monkfish not only good for you but also delicious.

2 Tbsp. avocado oil

4 butterflied monkfish fillets (4 to 6 oz. each)

2 c. fresh diced vine-ripened tomatoes with juices (about 3 medium tomatoes)

½ c. pitted and sliced Greek olives (about 10 olives)

2 Tbsp. freshly squeezed lemon juice

1 Tbsp. finely minced Italian flat-leaf parsley

Heat the avocado oil in a large skillet over medium-high heat, add fish the fillets and cook 3 minutes per side. (Monkfish cooks very quickly, so be sure to watch it carefully so you don't overcook it. You want the fish to still be tender and flaky!) Meanwhile, in a separate pot, add the diced tomatoes (and their juices) and cook for 3–5 minutes, or until the liquid is reduced by about half. Then add the olives and lemon juice and continue to cook for another minute or so. Then remove from the heat, and set aside. (Be careful that the ingredients at the bottom of the pot don't burn; add water as needed to prevent scorching the bottom.) When the fish fillets are done cooking, remove the pan from heat and transfer the fish onto plates. Cover each portion with the tomato mixture, garnish with parsley and serve hot.

Yield: Serves 4

Serving Suggestions: This meal is a lot to eat, but if you'd like to also have a side, you can add a vegetable like steamed broccoli or sautéed spinach.

PORTOBELLO BUFFALO BURGERS

Buffalo/bison meat is naturally lean and, if eaten as part of one's regular diet, has also been shown to reduce LDL (i.e., bad) cholesterol. It's also high in protein, iron, omega-3s and amino acids. Even better, buffalo are naturally disease-resistant and grow faster than domestic animals, which means that producers will typically raise them as naturally as possible, meaning without antibiotics and growth hormones. In fact, many of the unnatural (and very unhealthy!) techniques used to increase cattle (and other domestic livestock) production thankfully do not work for buffalo. Buffalo demonstrate what most of us have already known all along to be true—when it comes to our food supply, the less interference with Mother Nature, the better, for both the animals and our own health.

1 lb. ground buffalo meat, at room temperature (remove from the refrigerator at least 30 minutes before grilling)

1 Tbsp. paprika

½ Tbsp. garlic powder

½ Tbsp. onion powder

1 Tbsp. ground cumin

2 tsp. ground fennel powder

2 tsp. ground coriander

½ tsp. ground cloves

½ tsp. ground allspice

¼ tsp. ground black pepper, or to taste

4 large portobello mushroom caps (to use as burger "bun" halves)

a small amount of avocado oil, for spraying or brushing onto mushroom caps

toppings of choice: lettuce, tomato, red onion, red pepper rings, avocado slices, etc.

Preheat a grill to medium-high heat. In a large bowl, combine all the ingredients except the toppings and portobello "buns," mixing with a spatula until evenly distributed. Form into 4 (4-oz.) patties and grill for 2½ minutes per side, or until desired level of doneness has been reached. Brush or spray the portobello "buns" all over with oil, then simultaneously grill them next to the burgers, cooking them on both sides, until grill marks appear. Let the burgers and buns cool, then place the burgers onto the mushrooms with desired toppings and serve.

Yield: 4 burgers

Chef's Notes: If you've never had buffalo before, you'll probably be pleased to know that it doesn't taste gamey at all, nor does it have a strong flavor or aftertaste. It's really quite pleasant to eat. I would advise, however, that just as you would do with other lean cuts of meat (like London broil, turkey breast, etc.), you pay close attention to cooking times, as it can dry out if it's cooked for too long.

The nice thing is that these days buffalo meat is relatively easy to find. It's carried in a lot of generic supermarkets, so you won't necessarily have to go trotting off to a specialty store to find it.

WILD SALMON IN A SAVORY LEMON-DILL SAUCE

Fish:

2 (½-lb.) salmon filets (about 1 in. thick), with skins intact

1 Tbsp. avocado oil

2 Tbsp. finely minced garlic (about 4 large cloves)

1 large fresh bay leaf

2 Tbsp. water

Marinade:

¼ c. avocado oil

2 Tbsp. freshly squeezed lemon juice

2 Tbsp. paprika

1 tsp. ground black pepper, or to taste

¼ c. coarsely chopped fresh Italian flat-leaf parsley

2 Tbsp. finely minced fresh dill

Place the salmon filets and all the marinade ingredients into a large zip-top plastic bag, seal and gently massage the marinade into salmon from the outside of the bag. Refrigerate overnight. In a large (11–12-in.) grill pan, warm the 1 Tbsp. avocado oil on low heat and sauté the garlic and bay leaf for 5 minutes, or until tender. Add 2 Tbsp. water to deglaze the pan, scraping up any of the fond (the brown bits). Reduce the liquid by half, then the transfer fish fillets to the pan using a large spatula. Turn up the heat to medium and sauté the fillets, one at a time, for 3 minutes per side. When the fish starts to turn a light golden brown, check it with a knife or fork. The flesh should be soft but not too fleshy and easily flake from the skin. Discard the bay leaf. Remove the fish from the heat, transfer to a serving plate and let rest. The fish will continue to cook for a few more minutes as it's resting on the plate, so be sure not to overcook it. Using a sharp knife, divide the fish into 4 portions and serve immediately.

Yield: 4 servings

Chef's Note: It's much easier to cook each fish fillet whole and then divide into equal portions after you've finished cooking it. The skin will soften and be immeasurably easier to slice into. (Keeping the skin on during cooking will also help keep the fish moist.)

TUNA & AVOCADO LETTUCE WRAPS

2 (6-oz.) fresh albacore tuna steaks (about 1 in. thick)

2 Tbsp. avocado oil

1 tsp. freshly cracked black pepper

1 Haas avocado

2 Tbsp. freshly squeezed lemon juice

¼ c. diced celery

¼ c. shredded carrots

¼ c. pitted and chopped Greek olives (about 8 olives)

¼ c. sliced scallions, sliced crosswise into ¼-in. rounds

a few leaves of Boston lettuce (also called bibb or butter lettuce)

Place the tuna steaks and avocado oil into a large zip-top plastic bag, and then sprinkle the tuna all over with pepper. Seal bag and marinate overnight. Thirty minutes before cooking, remove the tuna from refrigerator and allow to rest until it reaches room temperature. Heat a large (12–13-in.) sauté pan over high heat until very hot, then place the tuna steaks into the pan and sear for 1½ minutes per side. Transfer to a clean plate (to avoid cross-contamination) and let rest for 10 minutes. (The tuna's internal temperature will continue to rise, cooking the steaks for another few minutes while they are resting.) Meanwhile, place the avocado and lemon juice into a large bowl and mash together until creamy. Next add the tuna and mash it into the avocado mixture until thoroughly combined, followed by the celery, carrots, olives and scallions. Divide the tuna into 6–8 portions and place each portion onto a lettuce leaf. Make into lettuce wraps: Place the stem side of the lettuce leaf facing you, fold down the top of the leaf toward the stem and then, holding down the top, fold over one of the sides and roll until lettuce is wrapped all the way around the tuna. Pin wraps with toothpicks, or tie together with green scallion stems, and serve.

Yield: 6–8 servings

COCONUT SURPRISE "CEREAL"

This breakfast dish serves as an option for those who might be missing cereal, yogurt or muesli in the morning. It's also far tastier than anything you can pour out of a cereal box!

1½ c. organic coconut milk

2 bananas, sliced

2 handfuls chopped walnuts

1 handful whole cashews

1 handful unsweetened shredded coconut

Combine all the ingredients in a bowl and serve.

Yield: 2 servings

SAFFRON-INFUSED COCONUT BARK WITH TOASTED ALMONDS & PISTACHIOS

½ c. sliced raw almonds

1 (13.5-oz.) can coconut milk

½ c. creamy almond butter

1 c. unsweetened shredded coconut

½ tsp. saffron threads

½ tsp. ground cardamom

½ c. shelled unsalted pistachios

Toast the almonds in a toaster oven at 350°F for 2½ minutes, being careful not to let them burn. Meanwhile, thoroughly combine the coconut milk, almond butter, shredded coconut, saffron threads and cardamom in an electric mixer and mix on low speed. Turn off the mixer and gently fold in pistachios and almonds with a spatula until well combined. Pour into a 7 x 5-in. metal baking pan lined with parchment paper, then transfer to the freezer and freeze for at least 2½ hours to solidify. Cut into bars and serve.

Yield: Makes 8 (2⅓ x 2½-in.) bars

NO-BAKE COCONUT-HAZELNUT BONBONS

These nutritious treats are perfect for busy athletes. They're healthy, portable, and extremely quick and easy to make. Eat them as pre- or postworkout snacks, or take them with you and just pop them in your mouth when you're on the go.

1 c. creamy almond butter

¼ c. chopped hazelnuts

1 c. coconut flour

¼ c. raisins

1 c. unsweetened shredded coconut

Combine the almond butter, hazelnuts and coconut flour in a food processor and process until ingredients are completely incorporated. Fold in the raisins and half of the shredded coconut using a baking spatula until well combined. Roll the dough into bite-size balls with the palms of your hands, then dip each ball into a small bowl containing the other half of the coconut flakes and roll around in the bowl to completely coat. Transfer each ball onto an 11 x 17 in. tray covered with waxed paper as you complete them, spacing them evenly apart from each other. Refrigerate to solidify. Eat and enjoy! Refrigerate any leftovers.

Yield: About 28 bonbons

Chef's Notes: If you're making these as a snack to go, just simply wrap them in small squares of waxed paper and place into an airtight container or large zip-top plastic bag. They also make great holiday treats as well. To give them as a gift, simply place the individually wrapped energy bites into a waxed paper–lined gift tin.

ICED COCONUT CHAI

Chai is a traditional Indian tea typically made by boiling tea leaves with milk, sugar and spices. This recipe has been inspired by that beverage, but has been revamped into a Paleo-friendly version. This recipe is made with coconut milk, which not only makes it extra creamy and delicious, but you also get the energizing, fat-burning benefits of its medium-chain triglycerides, too.

1 c. coconut milk

¼ tsp. ground cardamom

½ tsp. ground cinnamon

⅛ tsp. ground cloves

¼ tsp. ground ginger

⅛ tsp. ground allspice

⅛ tsp. ground black pepper

2 c. ice cubes

Combine all the ingredients in a blender and pulse until frothy and smooth. Serve immediately.

Yield: 2 servings (of 1 c. each)

PALEO VIRGIN MARY

The Virgin Mary is the non-alcoholic version of the Bloody Mary. This drink is a cool and refreshing accompaniment to dishes like barbecued chicken cooked on an outdoor grill.

4 c. diced vine-ripened tomatoes (about 5 large tomatoes)

1 c. coarsely chopped celery

1 c. coarsely chopped peeled carrots

¼ c. coarsely chopped scallions

2 tsp. ground pure white horseradish, or to taste (for medium heat, use 1½ tsp. instead)

½ c. freshly squeezed lime or lemon juice (about 2 limes or lemons)

¼ tsp. ground cayenne pepper, or to taste

½ tsp. ground black pepper

1 c. ice cubes

Optional Garnish Ideas:

4 large leafy celery stalks, cut in half

lime or lemon slices

carrot and/or cucumber sticks (use as swizzle sticks)

fresh basil leaves

red bell pepper slices

garlic, minced or crushed (mixed into the drinks)

Combine all the drink ingredients in a blender and pulse until smooth. Pour into a large pitcher and chill. Adjust the seasonings to your liking. Serve over ice cubes, decorating each glass with the garnish of your choice.

Yield: 40 oz., or 5 (1 c.) servings.

ORANGE SPICE TEA

All of the ingredients in this tea recipe have medicinal properties. For example, green tea has lots of antioxidants (and a lot less caffeine than other types of tea). Oranges have multiple health benefits: Their potent antibacterial properties help fight infection in the throat and get rid of chest congestion; their high levels of potassium can help provide relief from dizziness, nausea and fever; and their vitamin C content boosts immunity by increasing the body's white blood cell count, antibodies and interferon, which coats cell surfaces to ward off viruses and fight infection. Cinnamon has been shown to improve the body's glucose metabolism and lipid levels. And finally, drinking lots of hot liquids will help soothe your throat and rid your body of impurities.

4 c. water

2 whole Ceylon cinnamon sticks (about 3 in. each)

5 whole cloves

5 whole allspice berries

10 green cardamom pods

½ tsp. grated orange zest (from about 1 large orange)

¼ c. freshly squeezed orange juice (from a navel orange or other variety)

2 green tea bags

Bring a large pot of water to a rolling boil. Add the cinnamon sticks, cloves, allspice berries, cardamom pods, orange zest and orange juice, and continue to boil for another 6–8 minutes. Remove from the heat, strain to remove the whole spices and then pour into a tea pot or other heatproof container. (If it's easier, use heat-proof tongs first to remove the cinnamon bark before straining.) Immediately add tea bags, allow to steep for 1–2 minutes then gently strain and remove. Pour into tea cups and serve. Tea can be served either hot or cold (as an herbal iced tea).

Yield: 4 c.

Chef's Notes: If you'd like to make a big batch of this tea, simply quadruple the recipe, let it cool then transfer to a tall pitcher with a lid and refrigerate. This way, you can heat it up when you're in the mood for a hot cup of tea. Or, if you'd prefer it cold, just add ice cubes to the pitcher and serve. Be sure to make the ice cubes from the tea mixture itself, so you won't dilute the flavor of the tea.

Use a fresh orange when making the orange zest. The commercially sold dried orange peel is bitter and won't taste very good in tea. So, be sure to use the fresh stuff!

Also, use whole green cardamom pods (i.e., cardamom in its natural, unprocessed form) and NOT the bleached ones that are sold in many grocery stores. In the latter case, not only has their color been bleached out, but so has their flavor and nutrients! Natural green cardamom pods smell wonderfully vibrant and heady. And, when you boil the pods along with the other whole spices, they will make your whole kitchen smell absolutely divine! Green cardamom pods can be ordered online or found in a local ethnic (such as Indian, Asian, etc.) market.

FAQS

Q. What about a cheat day, week or month?

A. Trainers often tell us that the occasional cheat or treat does no harm when focusing on a healthier nutritional lifestyle. However, psychologically these words just reinforce the mistaken belief that healthy food is bland, unfulfilling, and something we eat only because we should do.

Think of "rich" food as foods that are abundant in nutrients, "treat" yourself to good quality foods that we were designed to eat and remember why "cheating" never works in the long run. There's always a cost, but there's no need to feel guilty about cheating, or like you're missing out when you avoid treats.

Q. What if I just can't find the time to exercise?

A. Instead of waiting for the right time or the right place, do what you can when you can. When you perform a movement repeatedly, your muscles become more efficient and improves your ability to perform this activity. Why not wake up in the morning and do some push-ups, or hang a pull-up bar at home and do a few chin-ups every time you leave the bedroom? Or hold a Hunter-Gatherer Squat (page 92) during television commercial breaks.

The key here is not to train to failure and to focus on the quality of the movement. This will still get you fitter and stronger and will add a significant number of reps without unnecessary fatigue and without a drain on limited time. Imagine if you were to do 10 push-ups a day when you wake up. That would equate to 70 push-ups a week and 3640 reps a year.

Q. I am concerned about failure! Anything I can do to stop feeling negative about this?

A. "No matter how many mistakes you make or how slow your progress, you are still way ahead of everyone else who is not trying."—Anonymous

Instead of thinking of not achieving an objective as failure, look at it as worthwhile education that will be useful for the next time you face this challenge. Decide what you can put in place to improve your prospects and stay positive by using affirmations. For example, instead of saying, "I want to give up smoking," say "I deserve to be and now enjoy being smoke-free."

Q. Is alcohol in moderation actually that big a deal?

A. Alcohol provides energy but is nutritionally void. There are significant social and peer pressures to drink and most of us are aware of the dangers of alcohol. Many of us justify and think of benefits to drinking and ignore any health issues as someone else's problem, or just us having to nurse a hangover once in a blue moon. However, if we take a view based on the acute impact to our health based on one night's drinking, our relationship with alcohol may change.

According to research, alcohol consumption is the cause of more than 60 different medical conditions, with 4% of all diseases globally attributable to alcohol.

Here are a few little-known facts about alcohol:

- Alcohol increases urinary calcium excretion and reduces Vitamin D metabolism (which may reduce bone density) and also reduces magnesium (which regulates and is essential for energy production) and phosphorous, low levels of which can lead to weakness in the shoulder and pelvic girdle muscles.
- Alcohol suppresses fat metabolism by up to 30% to 70%.
- Alcohol disrupts blood sugar metabolism by interfering with the regulatory hormones.
- Alcohol increases secretion of cortisol. Increased cortisol and decreased testosterone lasts up to 24 hours after drinking alcohol.
- Alcohol suppresses night-time spontaneous human growth hormone (hGH) by 70%, accelerating aging.

Q. Surely all those innovations in gym equipment must be for the better. Shouldn't we be looking forward and not backward when it comes to fitness?

A. Like most technology, some of the conveniences in the gym can be detrimental to our fitness goals. For example, running or walking on a treadmill will not provide the same physical and mental stimulation as performing the same activity outdoors. Most gym machinery is designed for isolating muscles and movement in a single plane of motion—repeating the same movement, in exactly the same path. This constant repetition and stress can lead to injury. Our bodies were designed to move across multiple planes of motion, and to work using multiple joints and using compound movements to perform tasks. For most people, working with your own bodyweight and utilizing everyday objects in your local outdoor environment to keep fit will provide the most benefit.

Q. Is going barefoot really better for us?

A. Shoes are a major cause of many foot ailments such as flatfoot and collapsed arches. They also change our natural gait and balance when walking, running and standing, causing many of the foot, hip, knee and back problems that plague us. Studies demonstrate that walking barefoot strengthens our feet and improves flexibility, posture and body alignment. Research has also shown there is a strong correlation between wearing running shoes and running injuries such as knee problems, ankle pain and shin splits.

Interestingly, the more support the shoes provide, the greater the likelihood of injury. One argument for why is that runners tend to avoid landing on the heel and instead land with a forefoot or midfoot strike. Avoiding the heel strike reduces the unnecessary forces and trauma suspected to lead to many running injuries.

To begin with, wear minimalist running shoes that provide limited support and work on strengthening the feet with barefoot drills, such as the Barefoot Walk Drill (page 70), and balancing exercises and movements such as the Squat (page 74). Be sure to start slowly; transitioning to barefoot can end up causing foot pain if your muscles are not slowly acclimated to the work. And always aim to move silently to reduce unnecessary stress on the joints.

Q. I can only work out indoors and have limited space. What can I do for an exercise like the Bear Crawl (page 94)?

A. As long as you have enough room to take one bear crawl "step" forward and then one "step" back to the start position, then you can repeat this movement, alternating sides on each crawl. You can use this in the confined space of a hotel room, or in a small apartment.

Q. What is a healthier substitute for my morning coffee?

A. According to a Chinese proverb, "It is better to drink green tea than to take medicine." Green tea contains much less caffeine than coffee and a whole host of antioxidants called phenols, including catechin polyphenols (catechin is the bitter taste of the tea), an antioxidant that raises resting metabolism by 4–8% more than coffee or water, thus it increases the effectiveness of your workout regime when used as a pre-workout drink.

Green tea has also been shown to reduce cancer risk, reduce LDL (bad) cholesterol, reduce high blood pressure and blood sugar, promote fat burning, reduce inflammation, preserve bone density and fight tooth decay, relieve stress and anxiety and fight against free radicals that can cause cell and skin damage.

The caffeine content in tea is minimal in comparison to coffee (14–24mg per cup as opposed to up to 200mg per cup for brewed coffee). I would restrict green tea to a morning drink to avoid any detrimental impact on sleep, and to drink it outside meal time to prevent any potential impediment of iron absorption.

Q. I sit down all day in the office. What can I do to address poor posture?

A. Take frequent breaks when using your smartphone, computer or tablet. Every 15 minutes, stand up, roll your shoulders and neck, pull your head back so your ears are directly over your shoulders, and avoid tilting your head forward. Go for a short walk if possible to improve blood circulation.

Q. Why do muscles ache sometimes after training?

A. Delayed-onset muscle soreness (DOMS) is a dull, aching pain with tenderness and stiffness in the muscles. It can feel uncomfortable but is a normal occurrence after unaccustomed or strenuous exercise. This can occur between 24 and 72 hours after activity. Some people rest altogether during this phase, but it's better to perform low-intensity work, such as walking, and maintain activity levels to increase blood flow to the muscles. It's necessary for muscle growth and adapting to exercise, and is an indication of previous activity that the body is getting used to.

Q. I want to convert my partner/brother/parents/friends to Paleo. It has worked for me and improved my health. But they won't listen! Any suggestions?

A. There has to be a desire and a need to change first. How many people smoke or binge-drink who are aware of all the dangers? It was 2 years before I was convinced by the Paleo argument. Seven years later I'm still happy with that decision, being fairly strict and with minimal adjustments from the basic principles since then.

What convinced me? It wasn't so much about evolution, or what our Stone Age ancestors ate. Firstly, it was about significantly improving the nutrient quota in whatever I ate while reducing the anti-nutrient load on my body. Secondly, if there were no manufacturing or processing of food starting tomorrow, what would I eat? It's unlikely I'd go to a wheat field and make flour, or find a cow to milk it, etc. Third, the improvements in my blood test results.

You need to find out what your friends or loved ones wants from their food. Then you can tailor your message to them, but only if they want to hear it.

Q. I am a social smoker and only smoke occasionally. What are the potential dangers?

A. Most of us are aware of the dangers of smoking, but only assume those who smoke heavily are at risk. Research shows that one cancer-causing genetic mutation can occur for every 15 cigarettes that a person smokes based on the cocktail of over 20,000 chemicals found in cigarettes.

Q. What about sleep deprivation?

A. Research from the University of Birmingham in the UK has found that just two nights of having two or three hours less sleep results in the body containing 15% more ghrelin (the hormone that boosts appetite) and 15% less leptin (the hormone that signals when you're full). This means you're more likely to be hungry based on a lack of sleep. A lack of sleep also increases the risk of obesity, type 2 diabetes, heart disease and hypertension. It also impairs immune system function.

A few tips to help you sleep soundly:

- Stop using electronic devices (smartphones, PC, tablets) 1.5–2 hours before bedtime. The light emitted from these screens can suppress melatonin in the brain, making you feel more alert when it is time for bed. If you have to use your PC before bedtime, reduce the impact by downloading free software f.lux (steropsis.com/flux), which adjusts the light from your computer's display based on the time of day and location.
- Keep the room dark and reduce ambient noise. Wear an eye mask and ear plugs if you have to!
- Avoid alcohol within 2 hours of bedtime, as although alcohol may make you feel drowsy, it reduces sleep quality and suppresses REM sleep, waking you up later in the night.
- Avoid caffeine within 12 hours of bedtime.
- Have a room temperature between 60 and 70°F. Our bodies are sensitive to temperature when we sleep, especially during REM sleep. If we're too hot or too cold, we generally become more restless.
- Avoid food within 2–3 hours of bedtime, as the digestive process may keep you awake.
- If you have to nap during the day, limit it to 20 or 90 minutes (not in between) no later than mid-afternoon so it doesn't affect your sleep at night.

Q. How does coffee affect my sleep?

A. Caffeine disrupts the quality of your sleep by reducing rapid eye movement (REM) sleep, the deep sleep when your body recuperates. You may believe that drinking a coffee in the morning won't have any impact at night, but the issue is that the half-life of caffeine is 6–8 hours. So even the 100mg caffeine from a cup of coffee first thing in the morning can affect deep sleep that night, as 25mg will still be in your system at bedtime (based on a 6-hour half-life).

RESOURCES

Ahern, Amy L. et al. "A qualitative exploration of young women's attitudes towards the thin ideal," *Journal of Health Psychology* 16, no. 1 (January 2011): 70–79, http://www.ncbi.nlm.nih.gov/pubmed/20709877.

American Physical Therapy Association, "Private Practice Section," accessed January 28, 2013, http://www.ppsapta.org.

Badrick, Ellen et al. "The relationship between alcohol consumption and cortisol secretion in an aging cohort," *Journal of Clinical Endocrinology and Metabolism* 93, no. 3 (March 2008): 750–57, doi: 10.1210/jc.2007-0737.

Baicy, K. et al. "Leptin replacement alters brain response to food cues in genetically leptin-deficient adults," Proceedings of the National Academy of Sciences of the United States of America, November 2007, http://www.pnas.org/content/104/46/18276.

Bastard, J.P. et al. "Recent advances in the relationship between obesity, inflammation, and insulin resistance," *European Cytokine Network* 17, no. 1 (March 2006): 4–12, http://www.ncbi.nlm.nih.gov/pubmed/16613757.

Batmanghelidj, F. *Your Body's Many Cries for Water: A Revolutionary Natural Way to Prevent Illness and Restore Good Health*, 4th ed. Tagman: Falls Church, VA: 2007.

"Beating Eating Disorders," Northamptonshire Healthcare website accessed January 29, 2013, http://www.nht.nhs.uk/main.cfm?type=NEWSITEMI&objectid=2914.

Bertolucci, L. F. "Pandiculation: nature's way of maintaining the functional integrity of the myofascial system?" *Journal of Bodywork and Movement Therapies* 15, no. 3 (July 20011): 260–80, http://www.ncbi.nlm.nih.gov/pubmed/21665102.

Björntorp, P. "Do stress reactions cause abdominal obesity and comorbidities?" *Obesity Reviews* 2, no. 2, (May 2001): 73–86, http://www.ncbi.nlm.nih.gov/pubmed/12119665.

Boutcher, Stephen H. "High-intensity intermittent exercise and fat loss," *Journal of Obesity*, 2011, http://www.ncbi.nlm.nih.gov/pubmed/21113312.

Bulhões, A. C. et al."Correlation between lactose absorption and the C/T-13910 and G/A-22018 mutations of the lactase-phlorizin hydrolase (LCT) gene in adult-type hypolactasia," *Brazilian Journal of Medical and Biological Research* 40, no. 11 (November 2007): 1441–46, http://www.ncbi.nlm.nih.gov/pubmed/17934640.

Calle, E. E. et al. "Body-mass index and mortality in a prospective cohort of U.S. adults," *New England Journal of Medicine* 341, no. 15 (October 1999):1097–105.

Calogero, Rachel M. "Objectification processes and disordered eating in British women and men," *Journal of Health Psychology* 14, no. 3 (April 2009): 394–402, http://www.ncbi.nlm.nih.gov/pubmed/19293301.

Cesvet, Bertrand. *Conversation Capital: How to Create Stuff People Love to Talk About.* Upper Saddle River, NJ: FT Press, 2008.

Cordain, L. "Cereal grains: humanity's double-edged sword," *World Review of Nutrition and Dietetics* 84 (1999): 19–73.

Cordain, L. et al. "Modulation of immune function by dietary lectins in rheumatoid arthritis," *British Journal of Nutrition* 83, no. 3 (March 2000): 207–17, http://www.ncbi.nlm.nih.gov/pubmed/10884708.

Cordain, L. et al. "Origins and evolution of the Western diet: health implications for the 21st century," American Journal of Clinical Nutrition 81, no 2 (February 2005): 341–54.

Cordain, Loren. *The Paleo Answer: 7 Days to Lose Weight, Feel Great, Stay Young.* Hoboken, NH: John Wiley and Sons, 2012.

Cordain, Loren. *The Paleo Diet: Lose Weight and Get Healthy by Eating the Foods You Were Designed to Eat.* Rev. ed. Hoboken, NJ: John Wiley & Sons: 2011.

Crabb, David W. and Suthat Liangpunsakul. "Alcohol and lipid metabolism," *Journal of Gastroenterology and Hepatology* 21, supplement 3 (October 2006): S56–60, http://www.ncbi.nlm.nih.gov/pubmed/16958674.

Dalla Pellegrina, C. et al."Effects of wheat germ agglutinin on human gastrointestinal epithelium: insights from an experimental model of immune/epithelial cell interaction," *Toxicology and Applied Pharmacology* 237, no. 2 (June 2009): 146–53, http://www.ncbi.nlm.nih.gov/pubmed/19332085.

Daniel, Kaayla T. *The Whole Soy Story: The Dark Side of America's Favorite Health Food.* Washington, DC: New Trends, 2009.

De Wit, B. et al. "Biomechanical analysis of the stance phase during barefoot and shod running," *Journal of Biomechanics* 33, no. 3 (March 2000): 269–78, http://www.ncbi.nlm.nih.gov/pubmed/10673110.

"Deaths from NDCs," accessed January 28, 2012, http://www.who.int/gho/ncd/mortality_morbidity/ncd_total/en/index.html.

"Department of Health: The Management of Adult Diabetes Services in the NHS," accessed January 28, 2012, http://www.publications.parliament.uk/pa/cm201213/cmselect/cmpubacc/289/289.pdf.

Diamond, Jared, "The Worst Mistake in the History of the Human Race," *Discover,* May 1987, http://discovermagazine.com/1987/may/02-the-worst-mistake-in-the-history-of-the-human-race.

Drago, S. et al. "Gliadin, zonulin and gut permeability: Effects on celiac and non-celiac intestinal mucosa and intestinal cell lines," *Scandinavian Journal of Gastroenterology* 41, no. 4, (April 2006): 408–19, http://www.ncbi.nlm.nih.gov/pubmed/16635908.

"Eating Disorders," National Health Services (NHS) website, accessed January 29, 2013, http://www.nhs.uk/conditions/Eating-disorders/Pages/Introduction.aspx.

Edwards, Darryl. "Nutrition: Is a Fruit Smoothie Better Than a Can of Coke?" *The Fitness Explorer*, last modified November 7, 2012, http://www.thefitnessexplorer.com/home/2012/11/7/nutrition-is-a-fruit-smoothie-better-than-a-can-of-coke.html.

Eliot, Lise. *What's Going on in There?: How the Brain and Mind Develop in the First Five Years of Life.* New York: Bantam, 2000.

Erickson, Kirk I. et al. "Exercise Training Increases Size of Hippocampus and Improves Memory." Proceedings of the National Academy of Sciences, January 2011.

"F as in Fat: How Obesity Threatens America's Future 2012." Trust for America's Health, September 2012, http://www.healthyamericans.org/report/100.

Fasano, A. "Surprises from celiac disease," *Scientific American* (2009), accessed December 8, 2012, http://www.scientificamerican.com/article.cfm?id=celiac-disease-insights.

Finkelstein, E. A. et al. "Obesity and severe obesity forecasts through 2030," *American Journal of Preventive Medicine* 42, no. 6 (June 2012): 563–70, http://www.ncbi.nlm.nih.gov/pubmed/22608371.

Francis, G. et al. "The biological action of saponins in animal systems: a review," *British Journal of Nutrition* 88, no. 6 (December 2002): 587–605, nih.gov/pubmed/12493081.

Fraser, A. F. "Pandiculation: the comparative phenomenon of systematic stretching," *Applied Animal Behaviour Science* 23, no. 3 (June 1989): 263–68.

Fraser, A. F. "The Phenomenon of pandiculation in the kinetic behaviour of the sheep fetus," *Applied Animal Behaviour Science* 24, no. 2 (September 1989): 169–82.

Frassetto, L. A. et al. "Metabolic and physiologic improvements from consuming a Paleolithic, hunter-gatherer type diet," *European Journal of Clinical Nutrition* 63, no. 8 (February 2009): 947–55, http://www.ncbi.nlm.nih.gov/pubmed/19209185.

Gershon, Michael D. *The Second Brain: A Groundbreaking New Understanding of Nervous Disorders of the Stomach and Intestine.* New York: HarperCollins, 1999.

"Global Health Risks: Mortality and burden of disease attributable to selected major risks," World Health Organization, 2009, http://www.who.int/healthinfo/global_burden_disease/GlobalHealthRisks_report_full.pdf.

"Global status report on noncommunicable diseases 2010," last modified Aril 2011, http://www.who.int/nmh/publications/ncd_report2010/en.

Hamilton, Marc T., et al. "Too little exercise and too much sitting: Inactivity physiology and the need for new recommendations on sedentary behavior," *Current Cardiovascular Risk Reports* 2, no. 4 (July 2008): 292–298, http://www.ncbi.nlm.nih.gov/pmc/articles/PMC3419586.

Harmon, K. G. et al. "Incidence of sudden cardiac death in national collegiate athletic association athletes," *Circulation* 123, no. 15 (April 2011): 1594–600, www.ncbi.nlm.nih.gov/pubmed/21464047.

Harris, W. S. "Fish oils and plasma lipid and lipoprotein metabolism in humans: a critical review," *Journal of Lipid Research* 30, no. 6 (June 1989): 785–807, http://www.ncbi.nlm.nih.gov/pubmed/2677200.

Heilbronn, L. K., and L. V. Campbell. "Adipose tissue macrophages, low grade inflammation, and insulin resistance in human obesity," *Current Pharmaceutical Design* 14, no. 12 (2008):1225–30, http://www.ncbi.nlm.nih.gov/pubmed/18473870.

Kay, A.D. and A. J. Blazevich. "Effect of acute static stretch on maximal muscle performance: a systematic review," *Medicine and Science in Sports and Exercise* 44, no 1., (January 2012): 154–64, http://www.ncbi.nlm.nih.gov/pubmed/21659901.

Kessler, David A. *The End of Overeating: Taking Control of Our Insatiable Appetite.* New York: Penguin, 2010.

Keukens E. A. et al. "Molecular basis of glycoalkaloid induced membrane disruption," *Biochimica et Biophysica Acta* 1240, no. 2 (December 1995), 216–28, http://www.ncbi.nlm.nih.gov/pubmed/8541293.

Klok, M. D. et al. "The role of leptin and ghrelin in the regulation of food intake and body weight in humans: a review," *Obesity Review* 8, no. 1 (January 2007): 21–34, http://www.ncbi.nlm.nih.gov/pubmed/17212793.

Kolaczynski, J. W. et al. "Acute effect of ethanol on counterregulatory response and recovery from insulin-induced hypoglycemia," *Journal of Clinical Endocrinology and Metabolism* 67, no. 2 (August 1988) 384–88, http://www.ncbi.nlm.nih.gov/pubmed/3292563.

Laitinen, K. and M Välimäki. "Bone and the 'comforts of life,'" *Annals of Medicine* 25, no. 4, (August 1993): 413–25, http://www.ncbi.nlm.nih.gov/pubmed/8217108.

Lieberman, Daniel E. et al. "Foot strike patterns and collision forces in habitual barefoot versus shod runners," *Nature* 463 (January 28, 2010): 531–35, http://barefootrunning.fas.harvard.edu/Nature2010_FootStrikePatternsandCollisionForces.pdf.

Majumder, K. and J. Wu. "Angiotensin I converting enzyme inhibitory peptides from simulated in vitro gastrointestinal digestion of cooked eggs," *Journal of Agricultural and Food Chemistry* 57, no. 2 (January 2009), 471–77, http://www.ncbi.nlm.nih.gov/pubmed/19154160.

McCaw, Steven T. and Jeffery J. Friday. "A comparison of muscle activity between a free weight and machine bench press," *Journal of Strength and Conditioning Research* 8, no. 4 (November 1994): 259–64.

McCusker, Rachel R. Bruce A. Goldberger and Edward J. Cone. "Caffeine eontent of energy drinks, carbonated sodas and other beverages," *Journal of Analytical Toxicology* 30, no. 2. (March 2006): 112–14, http://jat.oxfordjournals.org/content/30/2/112.full.pdf+html.

Mittlestaedt, Martin. "Canada first to declare bisphenol A toxic," *Globe and Mail*, August, 2010, http://www.theglobeandmail.com/technology/science/canada-first-to-declare-bisphenol-a-toxic/article1214889.

Moore, E. "Leaky gut syndrome: using probiotics and digestive enzymes in autoimmune disorders," *General Medicine* (2007).

Nakano, Y. et al. "A functional variant in the human betacellulin gene promoter is associated with type 2 diabetes," *Diabetes* 54, no. 12 (December 2005): 3560–66, http://www.ncbi.nlm.nih.gov/pubmed/16306376.

NCD Alliance, "The Global Epidemic," accessed April 2012, http://www.ncdalliance.org/globalepidemic.

"Obesity and Overweight" fact sheet, World Health Organization, published May 2012, http://www.who.int/mediacentre/factsheets/fs311/en.

"Obesity and the Economics of Prevention: Fit Not Fat," Organisation for Economic Co-operation and Development, published September 23, 2010, http://www.oecd.org/health/healthpoliciesanddata/obesityandtheeconomicsofpreventionfitnotfat.htm.

Oda, K. et al. "Adjuvant and haemolytic activities of 47 saponins derived from medicinal and food plants," *Biological Chemistry* 381, no. 1 (January 2000): 67–74, http://www.ncbi.nlm.nih.gov/pubmed/10722052.

O'Keefe, S. J., and V. Marks. "Lunchtime gin and tonic a cause of reactive hypoglycemia," *Lancet* 1 no. 8025 (June 1977), 1286–88, http://www.ncbi.nlm.nih.gov/pubmed/68385.

Okuyama, H. et al. "Dietary fatty acids—the N-6/N-3 balance and chronic elderly diseases. Excess linoleic acid and relative N-3 deficiency syndrome seen in Japan," *Progress in Lipid Research* 35, no. 4 (December 1996): 409–57, http://www.ncbi.nlm.nih.gov/pubmed/9246358.

Österdahl, M. et al. "Effects of a short-term intervention with a Paleolithic diet in healthy volunteers," *European Journal of Clinical Nutrition* 62, no. 5 (May 2008): 682–85, http://www.ncbi.nlm.nih.gov/pubmed/17522610.

Patel, B. "Potato glycoalkaloids adversely affect intestinal permeability and aggravate inflammatory bowel disease," *Inflammatory Bowel Diseases* 8, no. 5 (September 2002), 340–46, http://www.ncbi.nlm.nih.gov/pubmed/12479649.

Perrier, E. T. et al. "The acute effects of a warm-up including static or dynamic stretching on countermovement jump height, reaction time, and flexibility," *Journal of Strength and Conditioning Research* 25, no. 5 (July 2011): 1925–31, http://www.ncbi.nlm.nih.gov/pubmed/21701282.

Pleasance, E. D. et al. "A small-cell lung cancer genome with complex signatures of tobacco exposure," *Nature* 423, no. 7278 (January 2010): 184–90, http://www.ncbi.nlm.nih.gov/pubmed/20016488.

Price, Weston. *Nutrition and Physical Degeneration: A Comparison of Primitive and Modern Diets and Their Effects.* 8th ed. Price Pottenger Nutrition Foundation, 2008.

Ratel, S. et al. "High-intensity intermittent activities at school: controversies and facts," *Journal of Sports Medicine and Physical Fitness* 44, no. 3 (September 2004), 272–80, http://www.ncbi.nlm.nih.gov/pubmed/15756166.

Richards, Byron, and Mary Richards. *Mastering Leptin: Your Guide to Permanent Weight Loss and Optimum Health.* 3rd ed. Minneapolis, MN: Wellness Resources, 2009.

Richards, C. E. et al. "Is your prescription of distance running shoes evidence based?" *British Journal of Sports Medicine* 43, no. 3 (March 2009): 159–62, http://www.ncbi.nlm.nih.gov/pubmed/18424485.

Robbins, S. et al. "Athletic footwear affects balance in men," *British Journal of Sports Medicine* 28, no. 2 (June 1994): 117–22, http://www.ncbi.nlm.nih.gov/pmc/articles/PMC1332044/.

Room, R. et al. "Alcohol and public health," *Lancet* 365, no. 9458 (February 2005): 519–30, doi:10.1016/S0140-6736(08)61345-8.

Rudelle, S. et al. "Effect of a thermogenic beverage on 24-hour energy metabolism in humans," *Obesity* (Silver Spring) 15, no. 2 (February 2007): 349–55, http://www.ncbi.nlm.nih.gov/pubmed/17299107.

Sale, D., and D. MacDougall. (1981). "Specificity in strength training: a review for the coach and athlete," *Canadian Journal of Applied Sport Sciences* 6 (June 1981): 87–92.

Satoh, N. et al. "Sympathetic activation of leptin via the ventromedial hypothalamus: leptin-induced increase in catecholamine secretion," *Diabetes* 48, no. 9 (September 1999): 1787–93, http://www.ncbi.nlm.nih.gov/pubmed/10480609.

Schlosser, Eric. *Fast Food Nation: What The All-American Meal Is Doing to the World.* London: Penguin, 2002.

Schmidt, Richard A. and Timothy D. Lee. *Motor Control and Learning: A Behavioral Emphasis*, 5th ed. Champaign, IL: Human Kinetics, March 30, 2011.

Schmulson, M. J. "Brain-gut interaction in irritable bowel syndrome: new findings of a multicomponent disease model," *Israel Medical Association Journal* 3, no. 2 (February 2001): 104–10, http://www.ncbi.nlm.nih.gov/pubmed/11347592.

Schwarz, Barry. *The Paradox of Choice: Why More is Less.* New York: HarperCollins, 2005.

Sherwood, Lauralee. *Fundamentals of Physiology: A Human Perspective. 3rd ed.* Independence, KY: Cengage Learning, 2006.

Siler, S. Q. et al. "De novo lipogenesis, lipid kinetics, and whole-body lipid balances in humans after acute alcohol consumption," *American Journal of Clinical Nutrition* 70, no. 5 (November 1999): 928–36, http://www.ncbi.nlm.nih.gov/pubmed/10539756.

Simopoulos, AP, et al. "The importance of the omega-3/omega-6 fatty acid ratio in cardiovascular disease and other chronic diseases," *Experimental Biology and Medicine* 233, no. 6 (June 2008): 674–88, http://www.ncbi.nlm.nih.gov/pubmed/18408140.

Tabata, I. et al. "Effects of moderate-intensity endurance and high-intensity intermittent training on anaerobic capacity and VO2max," *Medicine and Science in Sports and Exercise* 28, no. 10 (October 1996): 1327–30, http://www.ncbi.nlm.nih.gov/pubmed/8897392.

Taheri, S. "Short sleep duration is associated with reduced leptin, elevated ghrelin, and increased body mass index," *PLOS Medicine* 1, no. 3 (December 2004): e62, http://www.ncbi.nlm.nih.gov/pubmed/15602591.

Temme, E. H., and P. G. Van Hoydonck. "Tea consumption and iron status," *European Journal of Clinical Nutrition* 56, no. 5 (May 2002): 379–86, http://www.ncbi.nlm.nih.gov/pubmed/12001007.

Thompson Coon, J. et al. "Does participating in physical activity in outdoor natural environments have a greater effect on physical and mental wellbeing than physical activity indoors? A systematic review," *Environmental Science & Technology* 45, no. 5 (March 2011): 1761–72, www.ncbi.nlm.nih.gov/pubmed/21291246.

Trapp, E. G. et al. "The effects of high-intensity intermittent exercise training on fat loss and fasting insulin levels of young women." *International Journal of Obesity* 32, no. 4 (April 2008): 684–91, http://www.ncbi.nlm.nih.gov/pubmed/18197184.

"Update on Bisphenol A for Use in Food Contact Applications," U.S. Food and Drug Administration website, January 2010, last modified April 2, 2012, http://www.fda.gov/newsevents/publichealthfocus/ucm064437.htm.

USDA National Nutrient Database for Standard Reference, last modified December 2011, http://ndb.nal.usda.gov.

Vaarala, O. et al. "Cow's milk formula feeding induces primary immunization to insulin in infants at genetic risk for type 1 diabetes," *Diabetes* 48, no. 7 (July 1999): 1389–94, http://www.ncbi.nlm.nih.gov/pubmed/10389843.

Virtanen, S. M. et al. "Early introduction of dairy products associated with increased risk of IDDM in Finnish children," *Diabetes* 42, no. 12 (December 1993): 1786–90, http://www.ncbi.nlm.nih.gov/pubmed/8243824

Wansink, Brian. *Mindless Eating: Why We Eat More Than We Think.* New York: Bantam, 2006.

Wolf, Robb. *The Paleo Solution: The Original Human Diet.* Las Vegas: Victory Belt, 2010.

Zarich, S. W. "Metabolic syndrome, diabetes, and cardiovascular events: current controversies, and recommendations," *Minerva Cardioangiologica* 54, no. 2 (April 2006): 195–214, http://www.ncbi.nlm.nih.gov/pubmed/16778752.

INDEX

T

U

V

W

Y